HEALTHY LIVING LIBRARY

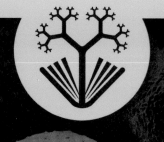

# BEYOND
# SEX ED

### Understanding
### Sexually Transmitted Infections

DIANE YANCEY AND TABITHA MORIARTY

TWENTY-FIRST CENTURY BOOKS / MINNEAPOLIS

Twenty-First Century Books™
An imprint of Lerner Publishing Group, Inc.
241 First Avenue North
Minneapolis, MN 55401 USA

For reading levels and more information, look up this title at www.lernerbooks.com.

Main body text set in Conduit ITC Std.
Typeface provided by International Typeface Corp.


**Library of Congress Cataloging-in-Publication Data**

Names: Yancey, Diane, author. | Moriarty, Tabitha, author.
Title: Beyond sex ed : understanding sexually transmitted infections / Diane Yancey, Tabitha Moriarty.
Description: Minneapolis : Twenty-First Century Books, [2024] | Series: Healthy living library | Includes bibliographical references and index. | Audience: Ages 13–18 | Audience: Grades 10–12 | Summary: "Approximately 20 percent of Americans have had a sexually transmitted infection. This timely and informative book outlines symptoms, treatment, and risk reduction practices for common STIs in the United States"— Provided by publisher.
Identifiers: LCCN 2022050965 (print) | LCCN 2022050966 (ebook) | ISBN 9781541588950 (library binding) | ISBN 9798765602300 (eb pdf)
Subjects: LCSH: Sexually transmitted diseases—Juvenile literature. | Teenagers—Sexual behavior—Juvenile literature.
Classification: LCC RC200.25 .Y348 2024  (print) | LCC RC200.25  (ebook) | DDC 616.95/100835—dc23/eng/20221122

LC record available at https://lccn.loc.gov/2022050965
LC ebook record available at https://lccn.loc.gov/2022050966

Manufactured in the United States of America
1-47458-48023-1/19/2023

# CONTENTS

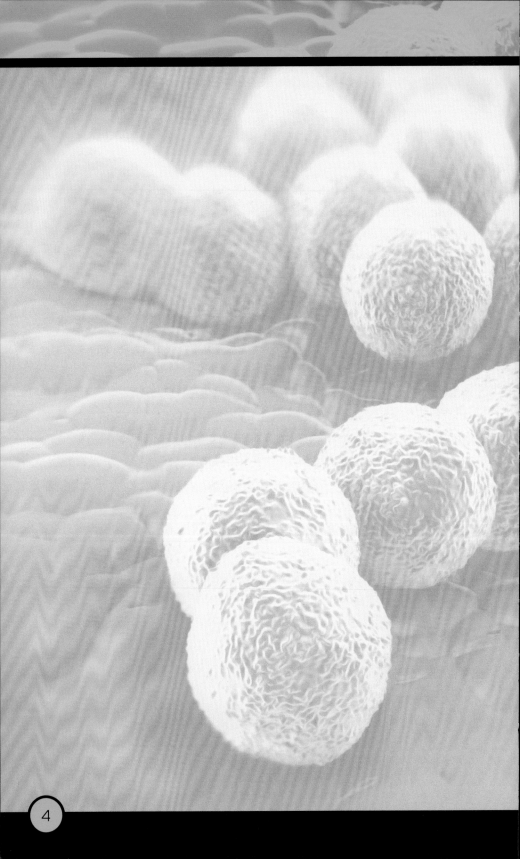

# A NOTE TO READERS

This book contains information about sex and anatomy. The authors acknowledge that while biological sex is fundamentally different from gender, these terminologies are inextricably linked in our society. Many people do not have a gender identity that aligns with the sex they were assigned at birth, and the language in this book may not accurately describe the reproductive systems of many others. Where possible, we have used gender-neutral language. When we discuss anatomy, the term *male* refers to the anatomy typical of someone who was assigned male at birth, and the term *female* refers to the anatomy typical of someone who was assigned female at birth. Additionally, many of the reported statistics related to sexually transmitted infections are categorized by sex. To preserve scientific integrity, we have not changed this terminology. We believe the terms *male* and *female* to be aligned with the patient-reported sex during data collection.

This book includes discussions about the risk of contracting sexually transmitted infections. The phrase *safer sex* is used throughout the text. Safer sex can mean many things depending on the aims and desires of the people engaging in sex. This book defines *safer sex* as sex where the parties are taking precautionary measures to reduce the likelihood of STI transmission. This may include using barrier protection, testing regularly, sharing information with one another about their sexual history, or any combination of these three.

# UP CLOSE AND PERSONAL

For many people, relationships are a top priority. The world would seem lonely without people to talk to, rely on, and love. But relationships, especially sexual relationships, can be complicated. The emotional and physical desires that arise while navigating the world of sex and romance can sometimes be bewildering and difficult to sort out.

Sexual feelings can be extremely strong during one's teens and early twenties, when many people begin to pursue romantic relationships or casually explore sexual relationships. However, it's important for people to think about their sexual values and boundaries before diving into this world. It can be easy to focus on feelings and desires and not consider the effects of one's actions. Sexual intimacy can be appealing, but it's critical to think about potential outcomes, such as pregnancy, curable infections, or lifelong illnesses.

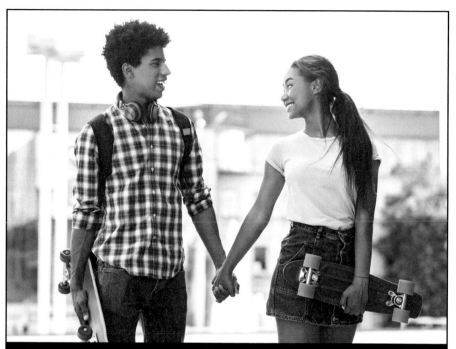

Teens and young adults in romantic and sexual relationships should be considering their physical and emotional well-being as well as that of their partners.

Sex can lead to sexual health problems such as sexually transmitted infections (STIs)—bacterial or viral infections that can be passed from person to person during intimate sexual contact. Medical professionals have identified more than twenty STIs. Some are rare in the United States. Others are common but, though uncomfortable, are not considered dangerous. Few STIs pose serious threats to public health in the United States. Still, STIs infect humans in record numbers, and some can be deadly or cause other deadly conditions such as cancer or liver failure if left untreated. According to the World Health Organization (WHO), more than a million STIs are acquired every day.

# CHAPTER 1

# WHY TALK ABOUT STIs?

**P**eople should be aware of STIs for a few reasons. STIs can significantly affect a person's health. An infection can impact fertility and increase the odds of developing cancer and other diseases. Some STIs can result in life-threatening conditions with few early warning symptoms. Knowing the symptoms of common STIs and understanding what to do if you suspect you are infected can make a big difference in health outcomes.

Understanding how STIs spread allows you to make choices to better protect yourself and your sexual partners from infection. Certain behaviors, such as having unprotected sex, can increase your likelihood of contracting STIs. Engaging in safer sex practices is one way to reduce the possibility of contracting an STI. But no matter what your risk level, it is wise to be well informed about STI transmission.

In the United States, young people are most likely among all age groups to contract an STI. In 2018 the Centers for Disease Control and Prevention (CDC), the top public health agency in the United States, estimated that one in five Americans had an STI. People between the ages of fifteen and twenty-four accounted for almost half of the twenty-six million new infections reported in the United States that year.

## I'm Infected *Where?*

One reason STIs continue to spread is that the diseases affect a portion of the human body—the reproductive organs, or genitals—that many consider to be very personal and private. Sometimes people will ignore a symptom they find and hope it goes away instead of going to a doctor because they are embarrassed to raise the issue. STI symptoms can also be hard to see. Many people do not regularly examine their genitals and may fail to notice a telltale blister or sore.

Familiarizing oneself with the human reproductive systems can improve the likelihood of identifying the symptoms or complications of an STI. It is often easier for a patient to communicate a problem with a doctor if they use medical terminology.

The next two sections describe the two types of human reproductive systems as male and female. The word *female* refers to the anatomy of someone who is assigned female at birth, and the word *male* refers to the anatomy of someone who is assigned male at birth.

## The Male Reproductive System

Most male reproductive organs are outside of the body. The primary sexual organ, the penis, is a tube-shaped structure made of spongy

# STI TRANSMISSION IN YOUTH

Young people between the ages of fifteen and twenty-four account for a substantial proportion of new STI cases. While individuals within this demographic may be more or less likely to acquire an STI based on their own sexual attitudes and behaviors, a few factors uniquely place youth at a higher risk than people twenty-five and older. These and other factors will be discussed in more depth in a later chapter.

- **Multiple sex partners.** People in this age group are more likely to have multiple sex partners than older individuals. "Multiple" could mean consecutive monogamous relationships or simultaneous relationships with different individuals.
- **Biology.** Studies have shown that young people with vaginas are more susceptible to STIs.
- **Barriers to health-care access.** Young people may not have health insurance or be able to travel to service providers.
- **Confidentiality.** Young people may lie to their doctor about being sexually active because they are afraid a parent or guardian will find out.
- **Insufficient screening.** Many young people do not pursue recommended STI screenings.

tissue and blood vessels with a smaller tube in the middle called the urethra. The urethra has a dual purpose: it carries urine from the bladder and male reproductive cells, or sperm, from the testicles

# THE MALE REPRODUCTIVE SYSTEM

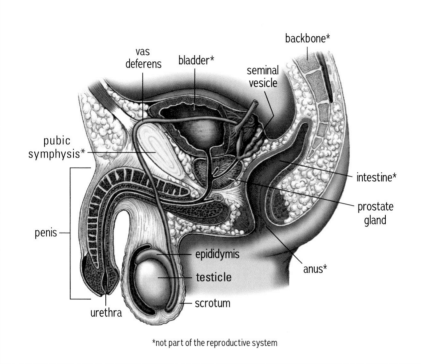

vas deferens
bladder*
seminal vesicle
backbone*
pubic symphysis*
intestine*
prostate gland
penis
epididymis
anus*
testicle
urethra
scrotum

*not part of the reproductive system

to the head of the penis and out of the body. When someone with a penis is sexually excited or aroused, the tissue of the penis fills with blood, and the penis becomes large and stiff, making it easier to insert into a mouth, vagina, or anus. Erections may also happen for no reason—this is the body's way of doing a "test drive" to make sure everything is working properly.

Two other primary reproductive organs, the testicles, lie behind and below the penis. They are a pair of egg-shaped organs encased

# SEX AND GENDER

Often people use the words *sex* and *gender* interchangeably, but they are different. A person's sex is usually assigned at birth based on the appearance of their genitalia but may also be assigned based on a combination of their chromosomes, hormones, reproductive anatomy, and other characteristics. Sex is often divided into male and female, but a person's hormones, chromosomes, or anatomy may not align with the usual definitions of male or female. In some such cases, a person may be intersex.

Gender is a social construct based on the societal norms, behaviors, and roles expected of individuals because of their sex assigned at birth. A person's gender identity describes how they perceive and express their own gender. In many cultures, gender has been understood as a binary—man and woman, masculine and feminine—but it is a spectrum of diverse expressions, experiences, and identities. Common terms used to describe gender include cisgender (self-identified gender aligns with sex assigned at birth), transgender (self-identified gender is different from sex assigned at birth), nonbinary (does not identify strictly with either masculine or feminine gender identities), gender-fluid (identifies with different gender identities in different ways day to day), and many others.

in a loose sac of skin called the scrotum. The testicles produce the hormone testosterone as well as sperm. Small tubules known as the epididymis and the vas deferens carry sperm from the testicles to the urethra. During ejaculation, sperm are transported out of the penis in semen. This fluid is produced by the prostate gland and the seminal vesicles. Both are located inside the body near the bladder.

The anus is the body's intestinal opening. It is located behind the testicles and the scrotum and between the buttocks. It is not technically part of the reproductive system but can be affected by STIs.

## The Female Reproductive System

Many of the female reproductive organs are inside the body. The vagina is a muscular canal that runs from the exterior of the body to the uterus. The vagina is a site of penetrative intercourse, and when someone delivers a baby, the vagina serves as the birth canal. The uterus is a pear-shaped organ that lies in the lower abdomen between the bladder and the large intestine. A fetus develops and grows in the uterus during pregnancy. The passage between the uterus and the vagina is the cervix, a smooth ring of connective tissue that softens or becomes more rigid depending on hormonal fluctuations. Set to either side of the uterus are the ovaries, where female reproductive cells, or eggs, and the hormone estrogen are produced. The fallopian tubes partially encircle the ovaries. A mature egg travels through them on its way to the uterus.

During birth, a baby passes to the outside of the birth parent's body through the vaginal canal. The external genital structure is the vulva, fleshy folds of skin and tissue called the inner and outer labia. The clitoris, an organ of sexual arousal, is externally about the size of

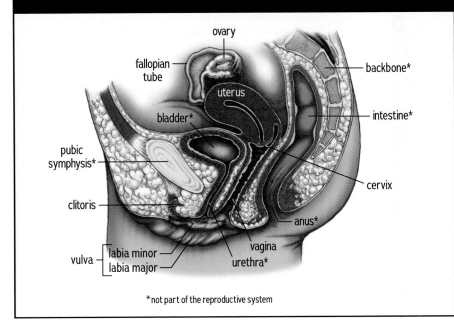

ovary

fallopian
tube

uterus

bladder*

pubic
symphysis*

clitoris

vulva — labia minor
labia major

backbone*

intestine*

cervix

anus*

vagina
urethra*

*not part of the reproductive system

an eraser on the end of a pencil and sits above the vaginal opening.
Internally, the clitoris consists of wishbone-shaped neural tissue
that extends between the uterus and the skin.

While the urethra and anus are not part of the female reproductive
system, they can both be affected by STIs. The urethra, through
which urine passes from the bladder, ends in a tiny opening between
the clitoris and the vagina. The anus is located behind the vulva and
between the buttocks.

# CHAPTER 2

# CHLAMYDIA

Caused by the tiny bacterium *Chlamydia trachomatis* (*C. trachomatis*), chlamydia is a very common STI that infects the urinary-genital area, the anal area, and sometimes the eyes, throat, and lungs. The CDC estimated that the United States had more than four million new cases of chlamydia in 2018. But this number is likely lower than the actual infection rate because many people who have chlamydia experience no symptoms and so do not seek testing. Various studies show that up to 50 percent of symptom-free individuals who are randomly tested for chlamydia test positive for the bacteria.

Chlamydia is especially common among young people, with fifteen- to twenty-four-year-olds accounting for two-thirds of new chlamydia infections each year. The highest rates of infection are among teens with cervixes. The tissues of the cervix are thinner for teens than for adults, making it more vulnerable to chlamydial infection.

## Transmission

There are many misconceptions about how chlamydia spreads. A common myth is that a person can catch chlamydia through kissing, sharing drinks with, or hugging someone who has chlamydia. Some claim that the bacteria can be passed on towels, toilet seats, bedding, or other inanimate objects. But this is not the case.

Chlamydia primarily infects the mucous membranes of the cervix and the urethra. It can also infect mucous membranes of the mouth, throat, and anus. Because of this, chlamydia is usually transmitted through oral, vaginal, or anal sex with an infected partner. However, chlamydia can also be passed from a birth parent to their baby as the infant passes through the vagina.

## Symptoms

People often don't experience any symptoms from chlamydia. They are usually surprised when they are told they have tested positive for the bacteria. A person can be symptom-free for life, or symptoms can develop weeks, months, or years after infection. Studies estimate that only about 10 percent of males and 5 to 30 percent of females ever develop symptoms. For those individuals who do have symptoms, they are usually mild and disappear about three weeks after exposure. But someone whose symptoms have cleared up can still be infected and transmit the bacteria to others.

Chlamydial eye infections produce conjunctivitis—redness, itching, and pain in the eyes. Infections of the anal area may include

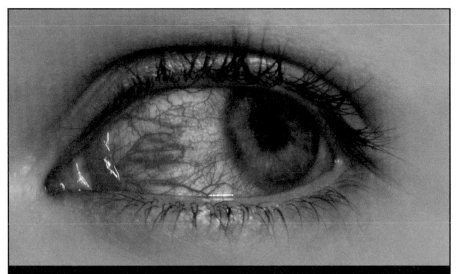

People often call conjunctivitis "pink eye" because it can cause the white of the eye to have a pink or red hue. Pink eye can be caused by chlamydia, but it can also come from other eye irritants such as allergens or contacts.

symptoms such as rectal pain, discharge, and bleeding. Some people develop reactive arthritis, a rare complication that involves recurring episodes of urethritis (infection of the urethra), arthritis, conjunctivitis, skin rashes, and other symptoms. This is the body's attempt to fight off infection by mistakenly attacking healthy tissues. Reactive arthritis may recur even after the infection has been treated with antibiotics. Reactive arthritis can be quite painful and can cause permanent damage to the joints.

A person with a penis may experience redness at the tip; a clear, thin discharge; burning with urination; and an itchy or irritated feeling in the urethra. In serious cases, a patient's prostate gland may be infected. They may also develop epididymitis, a medical condition involving inflammation of the epididymis. Epididymitis can lead to testicular pain, tenderness, and swelling on one or both sides

# DOCTORS AND CONFIDENTIALITY

When teens are asked during routine physicals whether they are sexually active, they may feel embarrassed or uncomfortable and answer no even if they are sexually active. Doctors speak to people of all ages about their sexual practices and sexual concerns, so there is no need to be embarrassed. They want to know if you have had any sexual experiences since your last visit so they can offer health services such as STI testing or birth control.

Doctors and other health-care providers can be good resources for teens who are uncomfortable talking to parents or other adults about sex. The relationship between a patient and a provider is completely confidential. But state laws differ on whether a doctor needs permission from a parent or guardian to administer certain tests or medications to minors. Parents who pay for their child's health insurance may receive a statement in the mail that lists the costs for the services received. Patients who feel unsafe disclosing their sexual health information to a parent or guardian can ask their physician what the privacy policies are for their office. They can provide information on how to seek a free

of the body. Scarring in the epididymis can result in infertility, or the inability to conceive a child.

Those with a vagina and cervix may experience a frequent need to urinate, burning during urination, genital irritation, and yellowish-green or low-cost health center that offers affordable care without involving insurance companies.

Some people might be afraid to talk with their parents about their sexual health. It can feel scary or intimidating, but usually it is a good idea to be honest with them. They will likely understand your concerns. Your physician can give you tips about how to talk to your parents about your sexual health or facilitate a conversation with you and your parents.

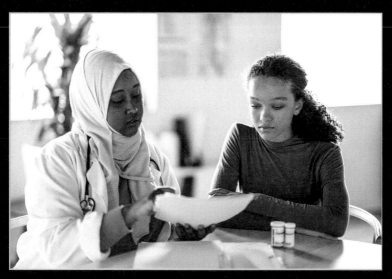

Having confidential conversations with a health-care professional can encourage teen patients to advocate for health needs they may feel embarrassed to ask about in front of a parent or guardian.

vaginal discharge. They may also experience inflamed cervical tissue that bleeds after intercourse. If chlamydia spreads from the cervix into the upper reproductive tract, it may cause pelvic inflammatory disease (PID). PID can be subclinical (with little to no symptoms), or it can be acute (causing abdominal and pelvic pain). PID can lead to scarring of the uterus, fallopian tubes, and ovaries. This scarring can lead to infertility. It can also increase the likelihood of ectopic pregnancies. Some people with PID may also develop perihepatitis, where the membrane covering the liver becomes inflamed. This can cause pain in the right upper quadrant of the abdomen.

A person can become infected with chlamydia repeatedly. These infections are usually more severe, with greater likelihood of PID. With each episode of PID, a patient has a 20 percent reduction in their chances of conceiving children, as well as a 20 percent increased chance of chronic pelvic pain and ectopic pregnancy.

Chlamydia can cause someone who is pregnant to go into early labor. About 30 to 50 percent of babies born to infected parents acquire chlamydial eye infections, and between 5 and 30 percent develop lung infections. For infants, such infections can lead to blindness, permanent lung damage, or death from pneumonia.

## Diagnosis

People should be tested for chlamydia if they have symptoms such as discharge from the urethra or vagina, a burning sensation during urination, or unusual sores or rashes on their genitalia. Even without symptoms, the CDC recommends getting tested if you have new or multiple sexual partners or have a partner with an active STI. They also recommend testing for people with cervixes who are sexually active and under twenty-five, as those individuals are more likely to contract chlamydia and have severe complications.

Someone may not be diagnosed with chlamydia until long after the initial infection. Since most people do not have symptoms, they may not think there's anything wrong or feel any urgency to get tested. Screening for chlamydia is not routine in people who are not part of one of the demographics with a higher rate of contracting the bacterium, so a doctor may not suggest testing for chlamydia if their patient has not confided that they are sexually active or that they are part of one of these demographic groups. The first time some people are diagnosed as having had chlamydia is often when they cannot become pregnant, after the fallopian tubes have been scarred by PID.

Several procedures are available to a person who decides to be tested for chlamydia. A health-care provider can help determine which procedure is best. The most sensitive and most widely used tests are nucleic acid amplification tests (NAATs). They analyze a vaginal swab or urine sample for genetic material from chlamydia bacteria. Similarly, enzyme-linked immunosorbent assay (ELISA) and polymerase chain reaction (PCR) tests, using blood and urine samples, look directly for the bacteria's genetic material. Doctors can also order a culture test, where a sample from the cervix, penis, throat, or anus is cultured (allowed to grow) in a lab. Lab technicians then look for chlamydia bacteria under a microscope.

## Treatment

Chlamydia can be cured with antibiotics, though they cannot reverse the aftereffects of PID such as scarring and chronic pain. For an uncomplicated infection, doctors generally prescribe an antibiotic for five to seven days. When the patient has PID or has an infected epididymis or prostate, doctors will prescribe an antibiotic for a longer period of ten or more days, depending on the severity of the infection. Patients should not engage in any sexual activities until they have completed their antibiotics treatment and their symptoms are gone.

# ECTOPIC PREGNANCY TREATMENT AND ABORTION CARE

An ectopic pregnancy is one of the most feared complications of conception. An ectopic pregnancy occurs when a fertilized egg implants anywhere outside of the lining of the uterus. The most common form of ectopic pregnancy occurs when the egg implants in the fallopian tubes. The first symptom of an ectopic pregnancy is usually pain. If the ectopic pregnancy goes

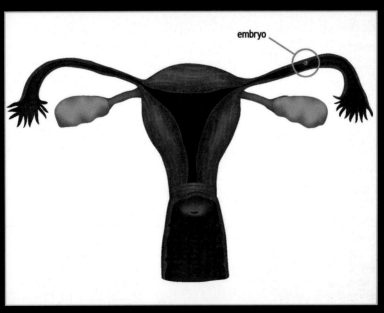

embryo

About 2 percent of all pregnancies are ectopic. A fertilized egg cannot properly grow outside the uterus. If an egg implants in the fallopian tube and is left untreated, it can result in a medical emergency.

untreated, the person may hemorrhage. In severe cases the fallopian tube may rupture, causing massive internal bleeding. These complications can lead to death.

Most ectopic pregnancies become life-threatening within the first eight weeks of gestation. Since the fetus is still too young to survive on its own and allowing it to remain means almost certain death for the pregnant person, the first-line treatment for an ectopic pregnancy is a medication abortion. These are performed by giving the pregnant person medications that halt cellular growth and block progestin, the hormone that maintains pregnancy. This terminates the pregnancy.

Some state laws restrict abortion at any stage of pregnancy. Since treatment for an ectopic pregnancy care is technically an abortion, pregnant people in these states may not have access to appropriate care for this medical emergency. Patients may have to travel to other states to receive the care they need. If unable to do so, they may suffer lifelong complications or even death because of this antiabortion legislation.

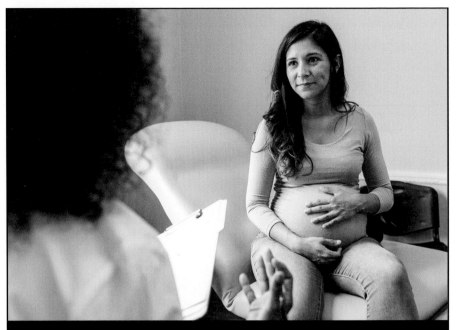

Testing and treating pregnant patients with STIs can prevent serious health complications for both parent and baby.

Pregnant people with an increased likelihood of contracting chlamydia and all pregnant people under twenty-five are tested for the bacteria at their first prenatal visit and during the third trimester. If a birthing parent is treated for their chlamydia infection, their baby is unlikely to be born with the bacteria. To help ensure that newborns do not develop chlamydial eye infections, hospitals routinely treat all babies' eyes with antibiotic ointment shortly after birth.

In many states, chlamydia infections must be reported to the state health department. This is because health officials focus on reducing and eliminating community spread, not just treating the person who tested positive for chlamydia. All people who have been partners of someone with an STI within the last sixty days need to be contacted about their potential infection. They are tested and, if positive, treated for chlamydia. In some states it is legal for health-care providers to give people with chlamydia extra medicine to give to their sexual partners. Follow-up testing is recommended for anyone who has received treatment so that the health department can make sure the infection has been eliminated.

# CHAPTER 3

# GONORRHEA

**G**onorrhea is another very common STI in the United States. It is caused by the bacterium *Neisseria gonorrhoeae* (*N. gonorrhoeae*). This bacterium can infect the genitals, mouth, throat, and anal area. In 2018 the CDC estimated that there were more than 1.6 million new gonorrhea infections in the United States. More than half of these infections occurred among young people between the ages of fifteen and twenty-four. Because gonorrhea is often asymptomatic, these reported cases likely represent only a small number of the new cases of gonorrhea each year.

## Transmission

Anyone who is sexually active can contract gonorrhea. It is transmitted through contact with the penis, vagina, mouth, or anus of someone who is infected. The bacteria are carried in genital discharge, semen, and vaginal fluids. Gonorrhea can also be passed from a pregnant person to the infant during childbirth. As with chlamydia, there is a myth that gonorrhea can be passed through contact with inanimate objects such as toilet seats and towels. This is untrue.

## Symptoms

Many people who contract gonorrhea don't develop symptoms. Any symptoms usually develop within two to ten days of sexual contact with a partner who has gonorrhea. Some people may experience symptoms as early as one day after infection, while others may feel nothing for several weeks. Symptoms can be so mild that they are often missed or mistaken for a urinary tract infection (UTI).

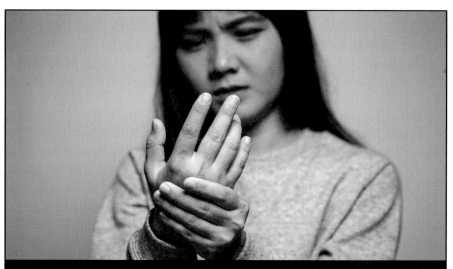

Gonorrhea can cause pain in the ankles, knees, elbows, and wrists. In rare cases, it can cause pain in the head and torso.

Symptoms of gonorrheal infection in the rectal area include rectal pain, itching, discharge, bleeding, or painful bowel movements. Gonorrhea of the throat, typically contracted during oral sex, may cause a sore throat. Redness and a thick yellow discharge mark a gonorrheal eye infection, most common in newborns. Very rarely, gonorrhea can spread through the bloodstream to other parts of the body. This can cause the rare and fatal disease disseminated gonococcal infection. Symptoms include fever, chills, joint pain, rashes, endocarditis (infection of the heart valves), and meningitis (infection of the lining of the brain and spinal cord). The most common symptoms of this condition are pain in the joints, pain in the tendons, and a rash.

Symptoms of gonorrhea in the female reproductive system may include pain or burning during urination, yellow or bloody vaginal discharge, or spotting between menstrual periods and after sexual activity. As with chlamydia, a gonorrhea infection can develop into PID. This can lead to internal abscesses, chronic pelvic pain, infertility, or ectopic pregnancy. Pregnant people who become infected with gonorrhea may experience miscarriage or premature birth. If gonorrhea is transmitted to their child during delivery, it can result in blindness, joint infection, or a blood infection that can lead to death.

In the male reproductive system, the most common symptoms are discharge from the penis and a moderate to severe burning sensation during urination. Discharge is usually yellow and heavy, although it can be clear and almost unnoticeable. Gonorrhea may also cause pain or swelling in the testicles. Complications from gonorrhea can include infection of the prostate, causing pain between the testicles and the anal area. If the epididymis becomes infected, scarring can cause infertility.

# ANTIBIOTICS AND RESISTANT BACTERIA

Penicillin, the world's first antibiotic, was discovered in 1928. Dr. Alexander Fleming of St. Mary's Hospital in London returned from a trip and found that one of his petri dishes had been contaminated with mold. He was going to throw it away and give up the experiment as lost, but he noticed that the bacteria he had been examining were dying where the mold was growing. After some testing, he realized that the mold was creating a chemical that killed the bacteria. He isolated this substance and named it penicillin.

A couple of decades later, penicillin was being mass-produced in the United States. For many years it was the first-line treatment for nearly every bacterial infection, including STIs. But doctors found that more and more bacteria that used to be easily killed off by penicillin were sticking around—even after multiple doses of the drug. Health-care workers switched to other antibiotics, but eventually some of those stopped working as well. The bacteria were becoming resistant to antibiotics.

The first way bacteria acquire resistance to antibiotics is through mutation. Most bacteria reproduce by duplicating their genetic material, or DNA, and dividing into two identical cells. It's common for errors to happen when copying DNA. Changes at the genetic level can impact the types of proteins a bacterium produces. Sometimes these proteins help the bacterium to be resistant to antibiotics.

The second way bacteria can become resistant is through horizontal gene transfer—the exchange of genetic material between bacteria. In this process, bacteria may swap sections of DNA. Sometimes the swapped DNA may provide antibiotic resistance to a bacterium that was not resistant before.

Using antibiotics can accelerate the rate at which bacteria adapt and become resistant. If someone uses an antibiotic, it will wipe out all bacteria that are not resistant—but it will not kill bacteria that have developed a resistance to treatment. These antibiotic-resistant bacteria then replicate and become more prevalent. The next time the antibiotic is used, it is less effective. Overuse of antibiotics can result in "superbugs"— bacteria that are susceptible to few or no antibiotics. Treating someone infected with a superbug is difficult or impossible.

Because of the threat of superbugs, researchers continue to search for new antibiotics. But this search is difficult, expensive, and often results in variants of antibiotics that already exist. "Since the discovery of new antibiotics is challenging," Chris Furniss, an antibiotics researcher at Imperial College London, explained, "it is crucial to develop ways of prolonging the lifespan of existing [ones]."

One way doctors try to do this is by advocating for antibiotic stewardship. Antibiotic stewardship focuses on only using antibiotics when they are necessary and using the smallest effective dosage for the shortest time to clear the infection. While this approach doesn't completely stop antibiotic-resistant bacteria from developing, it does slow their spread.

Research published by Furniss and others in 2022 revealed a possible new way to fight against antibiotic resistance: stopping the formation of proteins that make bacteria resistant. DsbA is a protein found in bacteria that helps fold resistance proteins into the right shapes to defeat antibiotics. The research team discovered that they could use chemicals to block, or inhibit, DsbA from folding resistance proteins correctly. "It is possible to reverse antibiotic resistance," Furniss said. "This means that the development of DsbA inhibitors in the future could offer a new way to treat resistant infections using currently available antibiotics."

## Diagnosis

The most common method of diagnosing gonorrhea is very similar to that of diagnosing chlamydia. A doctor can collect a urine sample or swab the urethra, vagina, or cervix and test using NAAT. Occasionally, a culture test is used for diagnosis. Unlike the tests for chlamydia, the Food and Drug Administration (FDA) has approved NAAT diagnostic tests to diagnose gonorrhea from samples taken from the throat and rectum.

## Treatment

As with chlamydia, health officials are concerned about gonorrhea and the possibility of community spread. In most states, gonorrhea cases must be reported to the state health department to ensure that all sexual partners of the patient are contacted and offered testing and treatment.

Gonorrhea can be cured with antibiotics. Sometimes gonorrhea can develop into a more complicated infection, such as PID or

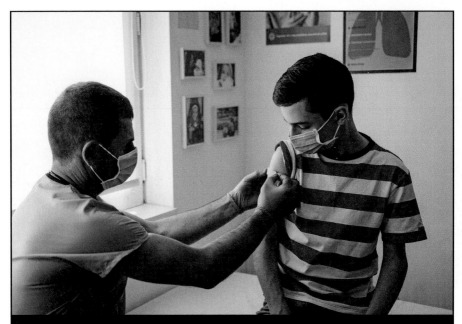

An uncomplicated gonorrhea infection can be treated with an injection of the antibiotic ceftriaxone.

endocarditis, when bacteria enter the bloodstream and grow in the valves of the heart. Then hospitalization or a longer course of antibiotic treatment might be necessary.

There are more and more cases of gonorrhea that are resistant to antibiotics. Follow-up testing is needed to make sure that the infection has cleared up. This should occur one to two weeks after treatment. When the infection is not responding to antibiotic treatment, doctors can prescribe alternative medications.

Follow-up examinations ensure that treatment has been fully effective. Reinfection is very common, so health experts recommend that people who have been treated for gonorrhea should return for additional retesting three months after their initial infection.

# CHAPTER 4

# SYPHILIS

Syphilis is caused by the bacterium *Treponema pallidum* (*T. pallidum*). Because of its spiral shape, the bacterium is called a spirochete. Known as the great imitator or the great pretender, syphilis can mimic a variety of diseases and can affect virtually every part of the body.

Some might think that syphilis is a disease of the past, but although syphilis was once on the decline, reaching historic lows in 2000 and 2001, numbers are increasing. There were 133,945 new cases of syphilis reported in the US in 2020. Men who have sex with men accounted for 43 percent of the syphilis cases in 2020. Some regions have higher rates of infection due to higher opioid use, lack of comprehensive sex education in schools, inability to access health care, or inability to access birth control. In 2021 in the US, there were more than 2,100 cases of congenital syphilis, where a pregnant person passes syphilis to their baby.

# Transmission

Like gonorrhea, syphilis is transmitted through sexual contact—
vaginal, oral, or anal—with a partner who has syphilis. Sources of
infection are syphilitic sores, rashes, and lesions and blood, semen,
and vaginal secretions. Bacteria enter an uninfected person's body
by passing through mucous membranes or through tiny breaks
in the skin. While the microbes are easily transmitted, there is
no evidence that syphilis can be transmitted on toilet seats; in
swimming pools, hot tubs, or bathtubs; by sharing clothing; or on
other inanimate objects.

When a pregnant person is infected, syphilis often infects a
fetus. Fetal infections can be very serious. Almost half of untreated
birth parents with a syphilis infection will have a stillbirth or will
deliver a baby that dies shortly after birth. Babies who survive have
up to a 70 percent chance of also having syphilis.

# Symptoms

A syphilis infection is divided into early and late stages. The early
stage of syphilis includes primary, secondary, and latent periods.
Primary syphilis starts at infection and lasts for several months.
The first symptom is a single, painless sore called a chancre. It is
small and round with raised edges. It appears between ten and
ninety days (the average is three weeks) after infection where the
bacterium entered the body. This can be the penis, scrotum, vulva,
vagina, anus, lips, or tongue.

Many people miss the initial chancre because it is painless and
is often in a hard-to-see area. Swollen lymph nodes in the genital
area may signal that something is wrong, but these are painless as

well and can go unnoticed. The chancre lasts three to six weeks and then heals with or without treatment. Even though the chancre has healed, the syphilis bacteria are still present. Because the chancre heals, the person might not seek treatment and may not know that they have syphilis.

Without treatment, secondary syphilis develops. During this period, bacteria enter the bloodstream and spread to other organs in the body. People are extremely infectious at this stage and have a higher likelihood of transmitting the bacteria through sexual contact. They can even pass the bacteria through nonsexual contact, such as through a cut or scrape in their or another person's skin. Symptoms may be like the flu and can also include

- a rash of brown sores, particularly on the palms of the hands and the soles of the feet
- swollen lymph nodes
- a sore throat
- weight loss
- joint pain
- a headache
- a fever
- hair loss

The rashes that appear during the secondary stage may even appear while the primary chancre is healing. They are usually not itchy. They can often look rough and reddish brown if they are on the palms of the hands or the bottoms of the feet. The rashes may also be very faint and difficult to notice. Some people also develop condyloma lata. These large, raised, gray or white lesions develop in moist and warm areas such as the groin, mouth, or armpits.

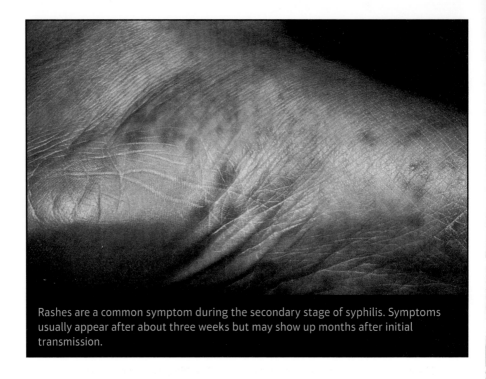
Rashes are a common symptom during the secondary stage of syphilis. Symptoms usually appear after about three weeks but may show up months after initial transmission.

If the disease is not treated at this point, symptoms disappear, and latent syphilis begins. This period can last for decades. When a person is in this latent stage, they are usually not infectious, and the infection can be detected only through blood tests. During this time, spirochetes multiply and spread into the circulatory system, central nervous system, brain, and bones.

A person with syphilis rarely reaches late stage, or tertiary, syphilis. Many people get treatment early in their infection, so their syphilis is eradicated before it progresses to tertiary syphilis. For those with long-term syphilis, 75 percent remain in the latent stage. They never show symptoms or progress to the next stage of the disease. If symptoms of tertiary syphilis do occur, they are extremely serious. Tertiary syphilis can damage almost any organ or system in the body. Neurosyphilis, infection of the nervous system, can cause progressive paralysis. Other symptoms include dementia, blindness, degeneration of the body's reflexes, vomiting, deep sores on the soles of the feet, and severe abdominal pain. Infection of the heart and major blood vessels can lead to death.

Some children born with syphilis may have no symptoms. Others may have a variety of problems that include failure to gain weight, fever, rashes, sores, bone lesions, and bone deformities. Complications such as deafness, blindness, bone pain, and deterioration of the central nervous system may appear later in their lives. Some characteristic signs of congenital syphilis include physical abnormalities such as a high forehead, the absence of the bony part of the nose (saddlenose), and peg-shaped teeth (Hutchinson's teeth).

## Diagnosis

Medical professionals have several methods of diagnosing syphilis. A doctor may recognize physical symptoms such as a chancre. They may swab lesions to obtain bacteria; then they are identified with a microscope. They may draw a blood sample and order blood tests. The most common blood tests are the venereal disease research laboratory (VDRL) test and the rapid plasma reagin (RPR) test. These tests will show a positive reaction within a few weeks of infection and will continue to do so unless an infected person receives treatment. They are quick and less expensive than other tests. But these tests may also react to other conditions besides syphilis, such as Lyme disease, pregnancy, malaria, tuberculosis, or systemic lupus erythematosus and other autoimmune disorders. So, when a VDRL or RPR test comes back positive, the doctor will order a follow-up test, commonly the fluorescent treponemal antibody absorption (FTA-ABS) test.

In many areas of the world, including parts of the United States, testing for syphilis during routine prenatal checkups is common. If a pregnant person is treated during the first four months of their pregnancy, the fetus probably won't be born with a congenital syphilis infection.

## Treatment

Most cases of syphilis, including congenital syphilis, can be cured with penicillin. But damage to the body's organs and systems cannot be reversed. For people who have had an infection for less than a year, an injection of penicillin usually clears up the bacteria. Long-term infections or people with neurosyphilis require a series of penicillin injections. Usually, doctors recommend that even people who are allergic to penicillin be treated this way after a short period of desensitization, when a patient is exposed to small amounts of an allergen over time to reduce the severity of their reaction. Penicillin is by far the most effective drug for treating syphilis. People with neurosyphilis who are allergic to penicillin are usually treated with another antibiotic, as neurosyphilis can be immediately life-threatening and the patient may not have time to undergo desensitization.

People do not develop immunity to syphilis and can be reinfected. So periodic checkups and regular testing are important. This is especially crucial in people who may also have an immune-compromising condition.

New cases of syphilis must be reported to a state health department to ensure that all sexual partners are contacted and can receive testing and treatment. Testing a patient's partners also allows a physician to determine if there is risk of worsening the patient's infection or of reinfection.

# CHAPTER 5

# GENITAL HERPES

Genital herpes can be a painful and disruptive part of someone's life. Caused by the herpes simplex virus type 2 (HSV-2), it is one of a family of viruses that causes cold sores, chicken pox, shingles, and mononucleosis. Herpes simplex virus type 1 (HSV-1), which causes oral herpes (cold sores), is a close relative of HSV-2. Oral herpes most commonly occurs around the face. It is transmitted through kissing. Oral herpes can also appear on the hands of someone who touches a cold sore. HSV-1 can also sometimes infect the genital area. HSV-2 commonly infects the genitals but can infect the face, the throat, and the eyes as well.

In 2018 the CDC estimated that about 572,000 new cases of genital herpes were diagnosed in the United States each year. About 12 percent—or one in eight people—in the United States between the ages of fourteen and forty-nine live with the virus. There are no known cures for herpes, but antiviral medications can help shorten the length of outbreaks and reduce the likelihood of transmission to sexual partners.

A study conducted in 2016 found that women were twice as likely to contract HSV-2 than men, likely due to anatomic differences. Among people with similar numbers of partners, HSV-2 infection is also more common among non-Hispanic Black populations than non-Hispanic white populations for reasons that remain unclear. Many people infected with HSV-2 are unaware of their infection because they never show symptoms and because asymptomatic people are very unlikely to transmit the virus. The CDC estimates that in the United States more than 85 percent of people between the ages of fourteen and forty-nine who have HSV-2 have never received a diagnosis.

## Transmission

Genital herpes is transmitted through contact with the actual herpes virus, which can be present in herpes lesions, the mucus membranes of the body, genital or oral secretions, and even skin that appears normal. Usually only HSV-2 is transmitted genitally, but someone can contract genital HSV-1 if they receive oral sex from someone with HSV-1.

After herpes is contracted, the virus migrates from the point of contact on the skin down the nearest nerve to a mass of nerve cells near the base of the spine. The virus can lay dormant (inactive) there for long periods. When it reactivates, it can travel through all the nerves that run out from that mass of cells. It then surfaces on the skin and mucous membranes, where it produces blisters and lesions. These can occur on the genitals, buttocks, groin, and the upper thighs.

Infected individuals feel perfectly healthy when they are symptom-free. But they will have periods of asymptomatic shedding. During shedding, the herpes virus is present on the skin and can be easily passed to others. Everyone who has genital herpes will shed at some point between outbreaks. A person cannot know when asymptomatic shedding is occurring, but experts find that people seem to shed most frequently just before and after outbreaks. During outbreaks, a person with herpes experiences symptomatic shedding and is very infectious.

Genital herpes can be transmitted from a parent with herpes to their baby during pregnancy, during childbirth, or shortly afterward. This type of herpes is one of the most dangerous complications of genital herpes. Herpes acquired at birth can be fatal to the infant and is one of the reasons why all people who become pregnant should notify their doctor if they have or think they have had herpes. New infections in the third trimester of pregnancy have the highest chance of transmission to the newborn, so pregnant people are usually counseled to avoid having intercourse with new partners or with any partners that are known to have genital herpes during this last portion of their pregnancy.

For the first few weeks of a genital herpes infection, before the body has time to build up immunity to the virus, a person can sometimes spread the virus to other parts of their own body. Called autoinoculation, this can happen by touching the infected area and then immediately touching another part of the body. This is an uncommon phenomenon. In people with weakened immune systems the virus can spread throughout the body, a process called dissemination. This, too, is rare. The sores caused by herpes virus can make it easier to transmit and acquire some other STIs, so people who are experiencing a herpes outbreak should take even more steps to protect themselves and their partners during intercourse.

The herpes virus is quickly inactivated when it dries. So it is unlikely to be transmitted on dry towels, toilet seats, and other inanimate objects. Herpes cannot be caught from sharing a hot tub or a swimming pool with an infected person.

## Symptoms

Some people who become infected with genital herpes never have symptoms and never know they are infected. Many others only have mild symptoms and may not recognize them as genital herpes. They may mistake their herpes symptoms for something else. For instance, they may experience pain during urination and think they have a bladder infection. Someone may mistake abnormal vaginal discharge for a yeast infection. They may use antibiotics or over-the-counter yeast medications and think they have successfully treated their problem because the symptoms go away. But the herpes infection has just subsided and has the potential to recur later.

If symptoms develop, they usually first arise within two to twelve days of infection. Initial symptoms may be a bump or red area and itching, burning, or tingling of the skin. These first symptoms occur during the prodromal period. They can warn a person with genital herpes that they are very infectious and are going to have an outbreak of herpes blisters. Genital pain or pain and tingling in the buttocks, hips, and legs also indicate that a person is going to experience an outbreak of blisters.

Not every person with genital herpes experiences prodrome. Many go right into the syndrome period. The most characteristic symptoms of the syndrome period are blisters, usually about the

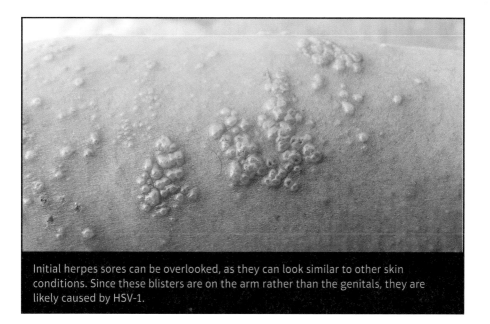

Initial herpes sores can be overlooked, as they can look similar to other skin conditions. Since these blisters are on the arm rather than the genitals, they are likely caused by HSV-1.

size of a pinhead (although they can be larger). They appear alone or in clusters. These can arise on the genitals, buttocks, groin, and anal area. They are often itchy and can be very painful. Tiny slits or painful ulcers can form when blisters burst. Blisters and sores that occur on skin surfaces usually scab over as they heal. Those that occur on mucous membranes do not.

Other symptoms of a genital herpes infection can include

- fever, nausea, chills, muscle aches, tiredness, and headaches
- difficulty and pain during urination
- swollen, painful lymph nodes in the groin
- weakness, pain, or tenderness in the lower back, legs, groin, and buttocks
- numbness in the genital area or lower back

Symptoms of genital herpes normally last five to seven days but may last up to six weeks. They may be so slight that a person never realizes they are having an outbreak. Or they can be very painful and traumatic. Some people miss work or school during an outbreak. Women with genital herpes tend to experience more severe symptoms than men do. Nobody knows why, but women experience autoimmune conditions at four times the rate that men do. These differences in immunity may also contribute to the higher severity of herpes symptoms in women. People with weakened immune systems generally have outbreaks that are longer and more severe.

In rare cases, genital herpes infections can become serious. The virus can inflame the lining of the brain and spinal cord, causing viral meningitis. Symptoms include high fever, stiff neck, increased pressure on the brain, and sensitivity to light. Viral meningitis can be life-threatening, especially when pressure on the brain is intense, but most cases clear up on their own. Oral herpes infections can cause encephalitis—inflammation of the brain—with headache, fever, and seizures. Newborns are particularly likely to experience severe health outcomes from the infection. Half of babies infected with herpes at birth die or suffer permanent neurological damage. Others can develop serious problems that affect the brain, eyes, or skin.

Genital herpes is recurrent—outbreaks can occur repeatedly throughout a person's life. Symptoms may seem to appear at stressful and untimely moments such as before a big test, at the beginning of a new relationship, or at the start of a new job. They may also appear at seemingly random times. On average, someone with herpes will experience four or five outbreaks a year, though some have eight or more. Over time, outbreaks usually become less frequent.

Experts do not fully understand what causes the herpes virus to become active, but various factors seem to trigger outbreaks.

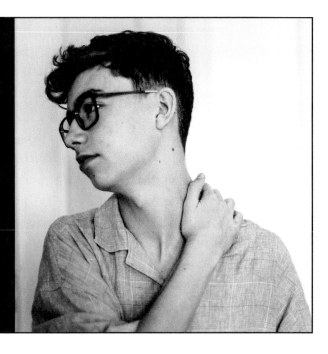

Most people recover from viral meningitis without treatment. But anyone experiencing meningitis symptoms should see a doctor.

These can include emotional and physical stress, fatigue, illness, and certain kinds of food such as nuts or chocolate. They might stem from hormonal changes during menstruation and pregnancy, poor eating habits, trauma to the skin, or exposure to sunlight. Although people with herpes can take preventive measures, and even if they do everything they can to avoid triggering the virus, sometimes outbreaks still occur.

## Diagnosis

Anyone who might have genital herpes should be tested as soon as possible. Delaying can make an accurate diagnosis more difficult. Those who suspect they are infected should stop having sexual contact until they know how to limit the possibility of transmitting the virus.

Several tests are available for genital herpes, and all must be performed by a doctor or another health-care expert. The most common and reliable is the lesion culture test. The doctor takes a swab or scraping of blisters or lesions and sends it to a laboratory for analysis. Antigen detection tests of material taken from blisters are also reliable. A positive result means that the genital herpes virus is present. A negative result may mean that no infection exists or that no virus was in the sample. When test results are negative but symptoms of herpes are present, doctors do a follow-up test to confirm the results. Both culture and antigen detection tests must be done during an outbreak.

Diagnosing dormant genital herpes through blood tests and laboratory analysis has been a problem for doctors. The ELISA test and the Western blot test look for antibodies to the virus in the blood. But the ELISA test does not distinguish between HSV-1 and HSV-2 infections, so patients who test positive won't know whether they have oral or genital herpes. The Western blot test is highly accurate in its results but is expensive and not widely available.

Because existing testing options are less useful for patients who aren't exhibiting symptoms, a standard STI panel will not include herpes. A doctor will only order a test for herpes if their patient has or reports symptoms. For these reasons, it is very important to specifically tell a health-care provider if you are concerned about herpes.

## Treatment

Genital herpes cannot be cured. Treatment can reduce pain and discomfort, shorten the outbreaks, and reduce the number of outbreaks. This is usually done through drug therapy and alternatives to traditional medicine. A doctor should be consulted for the best combination and course of treatment.

## DRUG THERAPY

Several antiviral drugs have been proven to shorten the length of genital herpes outbreaks. Antiviral drugs should be started within seventy-two hours of the beginning of an outbreak to be most effective and must be taken for ten days. Babies are at a much higher risk of developing severe complications of herpes because of their immature immune systems. If babies born with genital herpes are treated with antiviral medication immediately after birth, they have a much higher chance of avoiding the serious effects the disease may have when acquired at a young age, such as seizures, neurological damage, jaundice, and organ failure.

During the first year of infection, when outbreaks are often most frequent and severe, antiviral medications taken at a slightly lower dosage and for an indefinite time can reduce flare-ups. When taken this way, 80 percent of people have fewer outbreaks and 50 percent have no symptoms.

People who have herpes and take prescribed medicine can take several steps to maximize relief:

- Keep blisters and lesions dry to speed healing.
- Wear loose clothing for comfort.
- Get tested for other health conditions that may be weakening the immune system.
- Try a different antiviral medication if not getting satisfactory relief.
- Take the correct dosage of medicine as prescribed by a doctor.
- Identify triggers that may bring on an outbreak, such as stress, fatigue, and certain foods, and avoid them if possible.

# ANTIVIRAL MEDICATION VS. ANTIBIOTICS

While some antibiotics can kill bacteria that cause infection, antiviral medications do not kill viruses. They prevent viruses from replicating, or making more of itself. Viruses are unable to replicate outside of the host cell, so these antivirals can work a couple of different ways. Some antivirals may block the receptors the virus uses to enter the cell. Then it can't infect more host cells. Other antivirals might prevent the virus from replicating once it is already inside the host cells. And some antivirals boost the immune system, helping the person's body to fight off the infection. These methods help to reduce a person's viral load, or the amount of active virus in the body. With fewer active viruses, the immune system can more easily identify and fight off an infection.

Because all viruses replicate inside human cells, it can be difficult to manufacture drugs to harm the virus while not negatively impacting the human host. Most bacteria don't rely on host cells for replication, and even the ones that have their own replication machinery can easily be targeted with antibiotics. This difference in treating bacterial and viral infections is one reason why bacterial STIs such as chlamydia, gonorrhea, and syphilis can be cured and some viral STIs such as hepatitis B, HIV, and genital herpes cannot be.

## ALTERNATIVE TREATMENTS

Many people with genital herpes use alternative approaches to control herpes outbreaks, either with or instead of drug therapy. But some alternative remedies are expensive, some have not been proven safe, and many are not effective for most people. The following treatments may be beneficial, but a person should consult with their doctor before trying any of these:

**Stress reduction techniques.** Stress may trigger a genital herpes outbreak, although there is no scientific proof of this. But outbreaks can increase stress and make coping with symptoms more difficult. Counseling, regular exercise, relaxation exercises, meditation, biofeedback, or support groups for people with genital herpes can reduce stress, improve well-being, and help with other emotional aspects of living with herpes.

**Acupuncture.** This ancient Chinese practice of inserting small needles at certain key points on the human body can relieve a variety of conditions. While there are no scientific studies that prove acupuncture reduces the frequency of genital herpes outbreaks, some people with genital herpes say it decreases the pain during outbreaks.

**Nutrition and supplements.** Experts have proved that a nutritious diet helps support a strong immune system, which can make outbreaks of genital herpes less frequent and less severe. Some people believe that taking vitamin C, vitamin E, and zinc can boost the immune system. People with genital herpes who find that certain foods trigger outbreaks should avoid those foods.

**Tea.** Many people have found that damp black or green tea bags, placed on herpes sores, can be soothing. Soaking in a warm bath in which several tea bags have been steeped can be both relaxing and pain reducing for people with genital herpes.

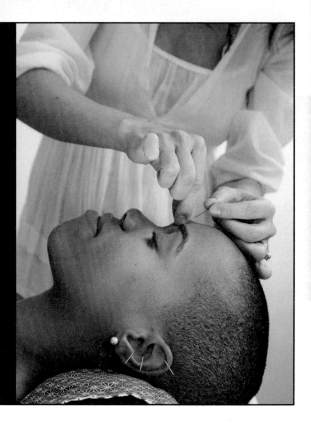

Research suggests that acupuncture can help with inflammatory skin conditions. This may explain why some people claim acupuncture helps in treating genital herpes symptoms.

**Drying agents.** Substances that dry the skin, such as cornstarch and rubbing alcohol, may promote healing of herpes lesions.

**Ice.** Cold compresses or ice, wrapped in a thin towel and applied to blisters or lesions, may lessen the severity of symptoms. Some people believe that ice can prevent an outbreak if applied during the prodromal warning period.

# CHAPTER 6

# HIV AND AIDS

**H**uman immunodeficiency virus (HIV) is the most complex of all STIs. This retrovirus attacks and weakens the immune system. At the end of 2019, the CDC estimated that about 1,189,700 people in the United States had HIV and that about 87 percent of them were aware that they were HIV-positive. While there is no cure for HIV, the infection can be managed with medication.

The immune system fights disease in several ways. It produces white blood cells. Some of them engulf and destroy worn-out cells, cancer cells, and pathogens such as bacteria, fungi, or viruses. Some white blood cells react to invading foreign bodies by forming antibodies, small proteins that attach to the invaders, inactivate them, and mark them for destruction.

When HIV invades the body, it targets two types of white blood cells, the helper T and regulatory T cells, which regulate the immune system by controlling the strength and quality of all immune

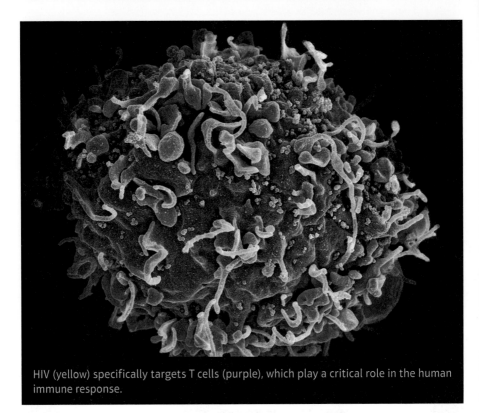

HIV (yellow) specifically targets T cells (purple), which play a critical role in the human immune response.

responses. HIV inserts its genetic material (the viral RNA) into the T cells, replicates inside the cells, and eventually destroys the cells as it goes on to infect others. When HIV first infects the body, a large amount of virus circulates in the system and T cell numbers decline.

The body's immune system is usually strong enough to suppress the virus for a time. At some point, the virus gains the upper hand, and the numbers of T cells start dropping significantly. Then a person's immunity becomes seriously impaired. A person who reaches this stage has acquired immunodeficiency syndrome (AIDS) and is at high risk of developing a variety of infections and diseases that can be fatal.

# RETROVIRUSES

Retroviruses are a family of viruses that replicates in the opposite direction that human cells do. Retroviruses have a genome made of ribonucleic acid (RNA). When a retrovirus enters a human cell, it converts its RNA into DNA and inserts it into the DNA of the human cell. The host cell treats this new DNA as part of its own genome, producing new copies of the virus. This type of replication makes it very difficult for the body's natural immune system to track down and fight retroviruses.

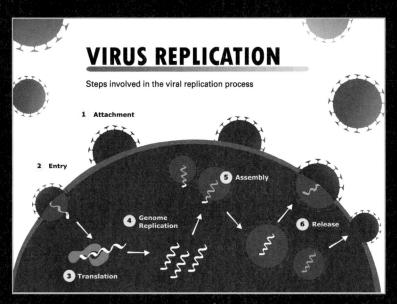

**VIRUS REPLICATION**

Steps involved in the viral replication process

1  Attachment

2  Entry

5  Assembly

4  Genome Replication

6  Release

3  Translation

To make new cells, human cells go through cell divison, a process in which the cell's DNA duplicates before the cell splits into two new ones that both have a copy of the DNA. By entering a human cell and replacing the DNA with its own, a retrovirus can replicate using the host's cell division.

53

While people of any race, gender, or sexual orientation can contract HIV, men who have sex with men are disproportionately affected by HIV and AIDS. This demographic makes up about 2 percent of the US population but accounted for 69 percent of new HIV diagnoses in 2019. People ages thirteen to twenty-four made up 21 percent of new HIV diagnoses in 2019, the highest of any age group.

## Transmission

Whether someone can transmit HIV to another person depends on their viral load. Someone with a high viral load has a higher likelihood of transmitting the virus than someone with a lower viral load. With treatment, individuals may have a viral load so low that HIV tests cannot detect it. A person cannot transmit the virus when they have an undetectable viral load.

HIV is spread in three ways: sexual transmission, contact with infected blood, and transmission from birth parent to child. Sexual transmission includes unprotected vaginal, anal, or oral sex or other genital contact where semen or vaginal fluids are passed between partners. The chances of becoming infected after one instance of anal or genital contact is between one in ten and one in three hundred, depending on a person's viral load. Parent-child transmission may occur through the placenta during pregnancy, through bodily fluids during childbirth, and possibly in breast milk during breastfeeding. Whether HIV can be transmitted through breastfeeding is unclear. The virus has been found in breast milk, but that doesn't mean the viral load is large enough for transmission. In cases where an infant contracts HIV from their parent, it is difficult for doctors to know whether transmission occurred before, during, or after birth.

Someone may contract HIV through contact with infected blood. Most often, this happens when people reuse or share needles. People who use intravenous drugs and share needles have a higher likelihood of contracting HIV than those who do not. Health-care workers are at particular risk for infection due to accidentally sticking themselves with a needle that has infected blood on it. But the risk is low, as health-care providers in the United States follow strict precautions for disposing of syringes and don't reuse them. Since blood banks began testing for HIV in 1985, the odds of infection from a blood transfusion in the United States have become very low.

HIV does not seem to be transmitted through casual contact. A person cannot transmit the virus by sneezing, coughing, breathing, hugging, shaking hands, or sharing work or home environments with other people. Even touching the urine, feces, or sweat of someone with HIV is unlikely to result in transmission.

## Symptoms

HIV often does not produce symptoms immediately after infection, although a newly infected person is highly contagious. If symptoms do occur, they can be mistaken for flu. They can include sore throat, fatigue, fever, headache and muscle aches, nausea and lack of appetite, swollen glands, and a rash over the entire body. Symptoms disappear after one to four weeks, and a person may not realize that they have HIV.

A period without symptoms follows initial HIV infection. This period may last many years. Individuals are not as infectious then as after initial infection or when AIDS develops. But people who know they have HIV and have a detectable viral load are still contagious and should make decisions accordingly.

# PREJUDICE AND THE AIDS EPIDEMIC

Before 1981 nobody had ever heard of HIV or AIDS. Then, in June 1981, the CDC reported 270 cases of Kaposi sarcoma in gay men living in New York and California. Kaposi sarcoma is a very rare but treatable cancer that affects the lymphatic system, so these cases alarmed the medical community. By the end of 1981, almost half of those who had developed Kaposi sarcoma had died. The number of terminal cases had medical researchers baffled and terrified.

Over the next few years, the CDC identified the previously unknown disease AIDS. By September 1983, they had determined that AIDS could not be contracted through casual contact, food, water, air, or by touching shared surfaces. But there was significant fear and misunderstanding about how the disease spread. Because of the concentration of cases among gay men, many people misrepresented AIDS as a disease that only gay men could contract, some out of ignorance and some intentionally. Religious and political authorities propagated stigma against HIV-positive individuals to promote their own antigay agenda, characterizing AIDS as a punishment for those who did not ascribe to heteronormative society. The LGBTQIA+ community suffered isolation, marginalization, and violence. Gay and HIV-positive individuals also faced discrimination in school, employment, housing, and other areas of their lives.

Thirteen-year-old Ryan White experienced discrimination due to his HIV-positive status. Ryan had hemophilia, a blood disorder that delays blood clotting. Usually, cuts and scrapes take longer to stop bleeding. But people with hemophilia sometimes need blood transfusions for loss of a significant amount of blood. Ryan contracted HIV during a blood transfusion. In 1985 his school in Indiana banned him from attending due to concerns that he would infect the other students. He and his mother fought for his right to attend. Even though scientific data had shown that HIV was not passed by casual contact, misinformation and discrimination prevailed. He was not allowed to return to his school. Ryan's family eventually moved to a new city, where the school body president led a schoolwide information campaign to destigmatize HIV and AIDS. Ryan was able to attend school, just like any other teen. He died from AIDS-related pneumonia in 1990, just before his high school graduation.

Governmental responses to the HIV and AIDS epidemic were slow, uncoordinated, and often insufficient. Funding for public health education and care for AIDS patients were particularly lacking. Near the end of the 1980s, some progress was made to address these shortfalls. In 1987 the first medication for HIV was approved. While it could not help those who had already progressed to AIDS, it slowed the progression of HIV and delayed the onset of AIDS. In 1988 Congress passed the first comprehensive AIDS legislation, known as the Health Omnibus Programs Extension (HOPE) Act. This legislation established protocols for AIDS research, established grants and programs to help states care for those with AIDS, provided funds for AIDS education and prevention programs, and specified

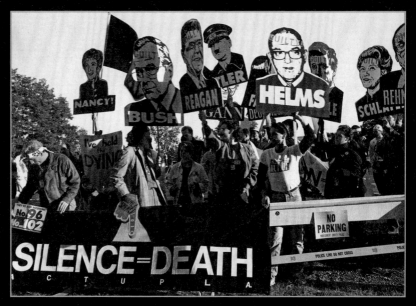

On October 11, 1988, fifteen hundred activists from around the US protested at the FDA headquarters in Rockville, Maryland. They demanded the FDA speed up research, development, and approval of drugs that could treat AIDS. Protesters held up signs of political figures with *GUILTY* written across their foreheads, including President Ronald Reagan, First Lady Nancy Reagan, and Vice President George H. W. Bush.

that all AIDS research should include data on marginalized communities such as people of color and LGBTQIA+ individuals.

The stigma and discrimination that ran rampant in the early years of the AIDS epidemic caused significant suffering and will not easily be forgotten by those who lived through it. HIV and AIDS receive less media coverage forty years later, but the physical effects of the disease and the stigmatization of those who have it are still prevalent in society. In his book

*Global Health Law*, Georgetown professor Lawrence Gostin writes, "So much has happened in the years since AIDS first emerged. Whereas once an HIV diagnosis was a death sentence, today patients can live long and full lives. But . . . [AIDS] remains a highly stigmatized disease. Remnants of discrimination can be seen everywhere, from the testing of health care workers and segregation of prisoners to travel restrictions and criminalization." One example of how HIV stigmatization persists is in discriminatory blood donation policies. The FDA bars men who have sex with other men from donating blood if they've had sex with a man within three months of their donation date. The FDA defends this practice with the claim that these men are more likely to contract (and therefore transmit) HIV. But donated blood already undergoes rigorous screening for HIV and other blood-borne diseases, and contaminated units are eliminated from the pool. If a man who has sex with men donated blood and it was HIV-positive, that blood would be eliminated with all the other contaminated units.

Over time, as the body's immune system weakens, symptoms reappear and eventually worsen. These symptoms include fatigue, shortness of breath, general discomfort, night sweats, persistent fever, swollen lymph nodes, diarrhea, and unexplained weight loss. The body's weakened immune system also allows a variety of mild infections such as thrush (a fungal mouth infection) and vaginal yeast infections to develop. Unlike earlier symptoms, these are usually severe enough that an individual will seek treatment. At this stage, people with HIV are very contagious due to a high viral load in the blood.

As the immune system fails, the body's T cell count drops. When a person's helper T cell count is 200 or lower, that person is considered to have AIDS. As AIDS progresses, infected individuals get sick with various opportunistic infections. These conditions normally are not life-threatening but can become deadly when a person has low immunity and cannot as easily fight off infection and illness. These opportunistic infections can include pneumonia, tuberculosis, herpes, fungal infections, Kaposi sarcoma, and non-Hodgkin's lymphoma (cancer of the lymphatic system). People with a cervix who develop AIDS are more likely to get cervical cancer as well as fungal infections, bacterial pneumonia infections, and progressive multifocal leukoencephalopathy, a viral infection of the central nervous system.

As AIDS progresses, illnesses become more frequent and more severe. Eventually, untreated people with AIDS are unable to recover from illness. They become thin and weak and cannot perform everyday functions. This decline is often slow and painful, and it can be a traumatic experience both for those with the disease and for those who love and care for them.

Children with HIV generally develop AIDS much more quickly

than adults do. The progress of their disease tends to be more rapid. Symptoms of AIDS in children are much the same as those in adults. But children also suffer from more bacterial, viral, and fungal infections than adults do. HIV infection can slow a child's growth and impair their intellectual development and coordination.

## Diagnosis

Medical professionals test for and diagnose HIV infection using a few different methods. An initial HIV test will usually be either a nucleic acid test (NAT), to look for the actual virus in the blood, or an antigen/antibody test, to look for both antibodies and antigens. These tests can detect HIV as early as ten days after exposure, so they are often used by blood banks to screen donated blood or to test babies whose birth parents are HIV-positive.

HIV can also be detected with antibody tests. Because it takes time for the body to produce antibodies, a reliable diagnosis cannot be made with an antibody test until three months after infection. A doctor may order an antibody test if a patient's HIV exposure was more than ninety days before or to confirm a positive NAT or antibody/antigen test result.

Doctors consider HIV to have progressed into AIDS if a person's helper T cell count has fallen below 200 cells per cubic millimeter of blood. (The normal level of helper T cells in the blood is about 1,000 per cubic millimeter.) If a person has an unexplained low white blood cell count, even if it is not below 200, and an opportunistic infection, one that usually does not cause disease in people with healthy immune systems, this can also lead to an AIDS diagnosis.

Viral load is also used to track the progression of HIV to AIDS. If a person has fewer than 10,000 virus particles per cubic millimeter

# WHAT SHOULD I KNOW BEFORE GETTING TESTED FOR HIV?

Deciding to be tested for HIV infection can be more difficult than deciding to be tested for other STIs. A lot of misunderstanding exists about what it means to have HIV, the way it can affect someone's daily life, and the kinds of treatments. Many people might delay being tested for HIV because they are worried about getting a positive result. The sooner a person is diagnosed with HIV, the sooner they can start treatment and reduce the likelihood of future health problems. Once someone has decided to get tested for HIV, they might ask a family member or close friend to come to the appointment for support.

Clinics, doctor's offices, hospitals, and state health departments typically offer HIV testing. Medical procedures carried out by a doctor or a clinic are confidential. This means they are part of a person's medical record and can be released only with the patient's written permission.

Some teens don't want their parents to know they're being tested for HIV, but in most situations, parents have

of blood, the viral load will be undetectable. An undetectable viral load does not mean the patient has no HIV in their blood. It does show that the patient's immune system is still working effectively. A patient with a high viral load has more than 100,000 HIV particles per cubic millimeter of blood. A high viral load can damage the patient's immune system, leaving that person open to opportunistic infections.

access to the medical records of minors. Teens can choose to take an anonymous diagnostic test that allows them to identify themselves only by a first name or a number. With an anonymous test, only the patient receives the results. An anonymous test can be performed in a clinic or with an at-home kit. Only an FDA-approved HIV home sample collection kit should be used for this.

Only one rapid self-test kit is currently available in the US, an oral fluid test. This kit can be purchased online or in most pharmacies. You can also purchase a mail-in self-test, which involves doing a finger stick at home and then sending in a dried blood sample. Free or reduced-cost HIV self-tests may be available near you. Contacting your local health department is a good way to find out about these opportunities.

Health-care providers can offer or direct patients who test positive for HIV to counseling or treatment. Additionally, the American Psychological Association has a web page with articles, webinars, blog posts, podcasts, and fact sheets that may help people as they grow accustomed to their new diagnosis.

## Treatment

Preventive care can greatly reduce a person's chances of getting HIV. People who are at a higher probability of acquiring HIV can use pre-exposure prophylaxis (PrEP). When taken as prescribed, PrEP is about 99 percent effective in preventing HIV infection. Some people have side effects from taking this medication, but they are generally

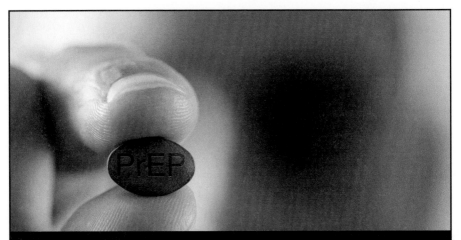

There are two pills approved for use as PrEP: Truvada and Descovy. Apretude is an injection drug that is also approved for use as PrEP. Each medication has different requirements and limitations, so patients should always confer with their doctor to determine which option is best.

mild and go away with time. PrEP is covered by most insurance plans and state Medicaid programs, and some other programs make PrEP available at little or no cost.

As of August 2022, two potential HIV vaccines are in clinical trials. One, developed by the pharmaceutical company Moderna, builds on the mRNA technology it uses in the COVID-19 vaccine. Another, developed by a biotech company, Excision BioTherapeutics, builds on technology that has been used for medications to strengthen the immune system as well as for gene editing. Both companies estimate that the first trials conducted in humans, which look primarily at the safety of the vaccine, will be completed by April 2023.

While there is not yet a widely available cure for HIV and AIDS, researchers have made many promising developments in treating HIV. In the United States, drug therapy, counseling, and lifestyle changes allow people with HIV to manage the disease much as they would any

# ARE WE CLOSE TO A CURE?

Five people are known to have been cured of HIV. They received stem cell transplants, some from bone marrow and some from umbilical cord blood and bone marrow. All the donors had rare genetic mutations that made them resistant to most forms of HIV. Since receiving the transplants, these five patients have recovered from HIV. Their bodies have eradicated the virus. One woman has been in complete remission from HIV after receiving immune-boosting treatments in 2006. While she still has HIV, her immune system has been able to suppress the virus without antiviral treatments.

Although five people have been cured, ethical issues prevent this type of treatment from becoming widespread. Receiving a bone marrow transplant is risky. The recipient's immune system must be completely suppressed before the transplant, and transplants don't always work. Because there are so many effective antiviral medications for HIV, doctors rarely advise patients to undergo the surgery.

Another ethical dilemma is that to confirm whether someone has truly been cured, they must stop taking their retroviral medications. Stopping and starting retroviral medications can increase the likelihood of antiviral resistance. If someone's medication is stopped and they aren't cured, they could end up with a more dangerous strain of HIV than they had originally. Finally, people with HIV resistance are rare, and bone marrow donation has its own possibility of complications. Bodily autonomy is one of the highest codes of medical ethics, and some worry that people with HIV resistance might be coerced into bone marrow donation.

chronic illness. But the drugs used to treat HIV are very expensive, and they are not always readily available in every country. For those without access to these treatments, the disease is still usually fatal.

## DRUG THERAPY

Management of HIV and AIDS is complicated and involves many visits to doctors or health-care facilities. Patients and their health-care providers must set up and manage individual medication plans. Regular blood tests are necessary to monitor T-helper cell and viral load levels and to see if medications are effectively suppressing the virus. Patients are also regularly tested for tuberculosis and, if they have a cervix, for cervical cancer. Any opportunistic infections must be treated and controlled to lower the odds of fatal complications. Because of such complexities, HIV treatment is lifelong.

An antiretroviral drug (ARV) treats infections caused by retroviruses such as HIV. ARVs work in different ways. Some block the conversion of the virus's genetic material from RNA to DNA. Others slow HIV by interrupting the release and function of new viral cells, rendering them noninfectious. Some other ARVs combat drug-resistant strains of HIV or prevent HIV from attaching to and entering human host cells.

Experts have found that combination therapy works best in treating HIV. When someone with HIV takes two or three drugs at the same time, the viral load can be reduced to undetectable and, therefore, untransmissible levels. Doctors usually prescribe a combination of ARVs as part of the highly active antiretroviral therapy (HAART) treatment. HAART is effective in stopping or slowing the progression of HIV to AIDS, prolonging the life and health of an infected person. But daily doses of medication can be up to twenty pills, and side effects are often severe. It can also be difficult to remember to take all medications correctly. Failure to follow instructions can allow HIV to become resistant to HAART treatment. Newer combinations of drugs may have multiple drugs combined into a single pill and have fewer side effects than older medications.

To get the best results from drug therapy, people with HIV should adopt preventive care methods as much as possible. This includes eliminating smoking, drug use, and excessive alcohol consumption. It also includes regular exercise and a balanced diet. Patients are also encouraged to follow safer sex guidelines to protect themselves against other STIs and to protect others from getting HIV.

## COUNSELING

Emotional support is a vital part of HIV treatment. A person may have strong feelings about their diagnosis. They may feel sad, angry, or anxious. They may experience strain in their relationships with

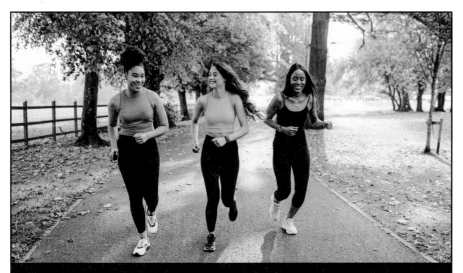

Regular exercise is a type of preventative care. Working out with friends can be more fun than working out alone and can help you stay accountable.

## TREATMENT COSTS

The cost of treatment for HIV, especially if it progresses to AIDS, can be extremely high. After years of treatment, totals can grow unmanageably large. In the United States, government programs such the AIDS Drug Assistance Programs (ADAP) help pay for costly medications for those who have limited finances or do not have private insurance. The ADAPs are state-run programs funded by federal grants. They are the primary source of expensive FDA-approved prescription drugs for those who can't afford them. The Ryan White HIV/AIDS Program, named after the teen who faced discrimination due to his HIV-positive status discussed on page 56, is a federal government program that financially assists people with HIV or AIDS who can't afford their care.

Various nonprofit organizations also assist those with HIV and AIDS who can't afford treatments. While ADAPs focus on providing drugs, groups such as the AAP-Food Samaritans help with other needs. This group provides monthly food vouchers to help improve quality of life.

family, friends, and partners after their diagnosis. Guidance and counseling from a psychologist, social worker, or health-care worker can make a huge difference in dealing with emotional distress, in maintaining a sense of hope and purpose, and in continuing to live a healthy life.

Traditional and online self-help, support, stress management, and grief management communities are available to individuals looking for additional resources. These communities can help

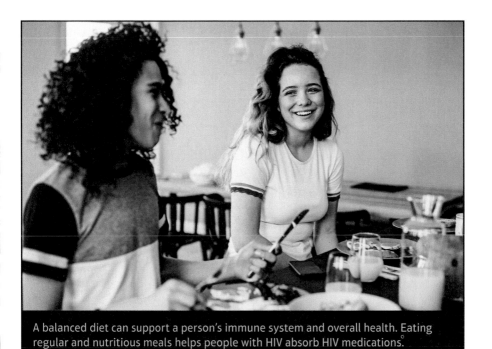

A balanced diet can support a person's immune system and overall health. Eating regular and nutritious meals helps people with HIV absorb HIV medications.°

someone learn to cope with the feelings and experiences that can be a part of living with HIV. Counseling centers and religious institutions also provide support and individual or group counseling.

## ALTERNATIVE TREATMENTS

Many people who have HIV combine traditional drug treatment and counseling with alternative treatments. These can include herbal therapy, acupuncture, massage, vitamins, and changes in diet. Practitioners of alternative medicine can provide advice and guidance in person or through online sites. Alternative therapies are meant to supplement, not replace, drug therapy. A person with HIV should consult a physician before pursuing these treatments to avoid potentially harmful interactions with their ARV medications.

# CHAPTER 7

# HUMAN PAPILLOMAVIRUS AND GENITAL WARTS

The human papillomavirus (HPV) is a family of more than seventy different types of viruses that cause warts on hands, feet, and genitals. Genital HPV is the most common STI. Most people have been infected with some type of HPV. Some kinds of HPV cause verruca vulgaris, or common warts that many people may have on their hands or feet. There are different types of HPV that are sexually transmitted and cause genital warts or cervical cancer. This chapter focuses on those types of HPV.

In 2018 the CDC estimated that about forty-three million people had active HPV infections in the United States and that thirteen

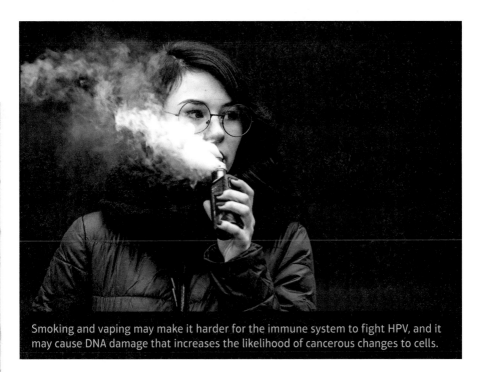

Smoking and vaping may make it harder for the immune system to fight HPV, and it may cause DNA damage that increases the likelihood of cancerous changes to cells.

million new infections occurred that year. Because HPV is so common, nearly every unvaccinated, sexually active person will get it in their lifetime.

Smoking or vaping may increase a person's likelihood to develop genital warts once they acquire HPV. Smoking and vaping suppress the immune system, allowing the virus a better chance to manifest itself. In one study of almost six hundred women, smokers were five times as likely to develop visible genital warts as were nonsmokers.

## Transmission

HPV lives in the skin and is transmitted through skin-to-skin contact. The most common way for genital HPV to spread is during vaginal, anal, or oral sex. A person can be infectious even if no symptoms are present, but the likelihood of transmission is greatest if contact is made with genital warts. The thin mucous membranes of the vagina, vulva, penis, and scrotum are particularly prone to infection. Babies can sometimes become infected with HPV at birth while passing through the birth canal of an infected parent. HPV is not passed through blood, semen, or other body fluids. Because transmission requires skin-to-skin contact, HPV can't be contracted from towels or other inanimate objects.

## Symptoms

Different strains of HPV have different symptoms. Most people infected with strains of the human papillomavirus that are more likely to cause cancer have no symptoms. Those who catch strains 6 and 11 (which are unlikely to cause cancer) and show symptoms typically see small warts that usually develop between thirty to ninety days after initial infection. In a few people, warts may not appear until years after the initial infection.

With HPV types 6 and 11, warts develop on the penis and scrotum, inside the urethra, around and inside the vagina, and on the cervix. They may appear inside and around the anus, on the lower abdomen and upper thighs, and in the groin. Occasionally, they occur in the mouth and throat or on the lips, eyelids, and nipples. A person may never know they have genital warts if they only appear in hard-to-see areas, such as inside the urethra, on the walls of the vagina, or on the cervix.

Genital warts can look like regular warts. They may be flesh colored or darker, and they are usually harder than surrounding tissue. They may be flat or raised, single or multiple, large or small.

They can grow, spread, and assume a cauliflower-like appearance, or they may remain small and barely noticeable. They may itch, but they usually do not hurt unless they are scratched and become irritated. Often genital warts go away without treatment. But the virus does not necessarily disappear. It can remain in the body indefinitely, and when it reactivates, new outbreaks of warts can occur. People can experience outbreaks of genital warts throughout their life, although the virus usually becomes less active with time.

Certain types of genital HPV are less likely to cause genital warts but increase the chances of developing cancer in infected areas, particularly cancers of the penis, anus, throat, vulva, and cervix.

According to the American Cancer Society, about fourteen thousand women develop cervical cancer every year, and about four thousand of them die from it even with screening and treatment. HPV types 16, 18, 31, and 33 have been found to be responsible for cellular changes that can lead to cervical cancer. When cervical cancer lesions are examined under a microscope, HPV is detected almost 100 percent of the time.

Genital warts can also cause problems during pregnancy, when they tend to grow rapidly. If they enlarge, they can make urination difficult. If present on the wall of the vagina, they can cause obstruction during childbirth. Infants exposed to HPV during childbirth may develop warts on their larynx, or voice box. This potentially life-threatening condition requires multiple surgeries to keep the baby's airways open.

## Diagnosis

Most people who have HPV never know that they have it because they do not develop any symptoms. HPV is almost always diagnosed by the presence of visible warts. People who suspect they may have genital warts need to be seen and diagnosed by an experienced health-care provider. The skin of the genitals is often naturally bumpy and irregular. A trained, professional eye can decide what is normal.

HPV is linked to several types of cancer, most commonly cervical cancer. A person may find out they have HPV through a regular cervical cancer screening procedure called a Pap test. A Pap test is performed during a normal gynecological exam. A physician places a device called a speculum into the vagina and opens it to visually inspect the cervix. Then the physician uses a plastic brush to collect cells from the transformation zone of the cervix, a place where two different types of cells meet. The transformation zone is the most common location for cervical cancer to arise. This plastic brush is placed in a medium to preserve the cells and sent to a lab where a pathologist looks at the cells to see if they have any abnormalities and might indicate cancer or precancerous lesions. HPV is the number one cause of cervical cancer, so precancerous changes of cells are usually due to HPV or, occasionally, other environmental factors. The Pap test is not a diagnostic tool for HPV or other STIs since it only looks for abnormal cells that might indicate cancer, although often when somebody has an abnormal Pap test it is due to HPV. A person can have a normal Pap test and still be infected with HPV or other STIs.

An abnormal Pap test result often leads to additional testing. If the patient is thirty years old or older, their doctor may call for an HPV test. It detects HPV strains that put a person at high risk of developing cervical cancer. It is not used as a general test for HPV.

A doctor may also recommend a colposcopy to closely inspect the cervix with a bright light and a magnifying instrument called

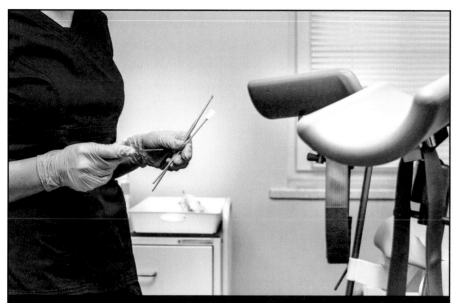

Generally, doctors recommend that patients with cervixes begin getting Pap tests at age twenty-one and continue to get regular Pap tests every three years. This recommendation may vary depending on a patient's personal or family history of cervical cancer.

a colposcope. A colposcopy can help detect HPV by allowing the doctor to see otherwise hard-to-see warts.

## Treatment

The HPV vaccine teaches the body to respond to HPV infections so that the immune system will be able to clear the virus quickly. Receiving the vaccine makes it much less likely for a person to develop HPV-related cancers in the future. Douglas R. Lowy, acting director of the National Cancer Institute, said at a conference in 2022 that "several countries which adopted HPV vaccination on a nationwide basis are showing that women who were vaccinated

# MONKEYPOX

On August 4, 2022, the US declared monkeypox to be a public health emergency. The virus is endemic to West Africa but early in 2022 began to spread throughout Europe and North America, where it was previously uncommon. The virus was also spreading in a different way than in the past—through sexual contact.

Monkeypox is related to smallpox but is less deadly and disfiguring. The main complication that most people experience from monkeypox is a very painful rash. It is spread through close and prolonged physical contact with infected skin.

The virus initially spread among men who have sex with men, which many people have used to justify stigma and bias around monkeypox. But just because the virus has spread in this population does not mean that it can't spread in other populations. Anyone who has contact with a monkeypox rash may contract the virus, regardless of sex, gender, or sexual orientation.

A few antiviral medications treat severe cases of monkeypox. The most prevalent is TPOXX, an antiviral that was initially approved to treat smallpox but was developed through testing on monkeypox. Some vaccines are available

when they were sixteen years or younger—this is in Denmark—have about a 90 percent decrease in their development of cervical cancer." The vaccine is recommended for individuals between the ages of eleven and twenty-six. Because the vaccine protects against for people who are at higher likelihood of contracting monkeypox, such as those who have compromised immune systems and men who have sex with men.

Although monkeypox has not historically been considered an STI, it is functioning as one. At the time of this book's printing, it remains to be seen whether monkeypox will continue to spread as an STI or regress to its less prevalent form.

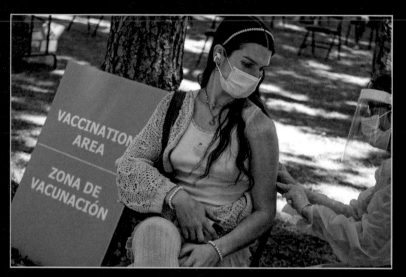

A Medical Reserve Corps volunteer administers a monkeypox vaccination at a walk-up vaccination site in Hollywood, California.

new infections but does not treat existing infections, doctors do not usually recommend vaccination for older patients who likely have been exposed to HPV.

There is currently no cure for HPV. Because most types of genital warts are not dangerous, some people choose not to seek treatment and see if they go away on their own. Often they do. But others choose to have genital warts removed, especially if they are large, irritated, bleeding, or embarrassing.

Medical professionals have several procedures for removing genital warts. Depending on the size, number, and location of the growths, different procedures may be more effective. These include

- cryotherapy—freezing and destroying wart tissue with liquid nitrogen
- physician-applied medications such as podophyllin and trichloroacetic acid that destroy the wart tissue
- prescription medications such as imiquimod cream that encourage an immune response to the wart
- electrocautery or laser therapy—burning and destroying wart tissue using electricity or lasers
- surgical removal
- interferon alfa treatment—protein injections that encourage an immune response to the wart

These treatments can eliminate warts and may lower the likelihood of transmitting the virus to others. But removal does not guarantee that the warts will permanently disappear. Most people who have genital warts removed will experience recurrences.

# CHAPTER 8

# HEPATITIS B

Hepatitis B is one of a family of hepatitis viruses. Unlike hepatitis A, which is spread through contaminated food and water, hepatitis B is commonly passed through an exchange of infected body fluids. Hepatitis C is a blood-borne strain that is usually transmitted through sharing needles but, in rare cases, can be transmitted through sexual contact. In the United States, hepatitis A, B, and C are the most common types. Other strains of the disease are hepatitis D (blood-borne) and E (commonly spread through contaminated drinking water). Both are rare in the United States.

Effective vaccines are available for hepatitis A and B. Even though the vaccine for hepatitis B has lowered rates of transmission, the CDC still estimates that there were 22,600 new hepatitis B cases in the United States in 2018. The reported rate of new infections is highest in adults twenty to forty-nine.

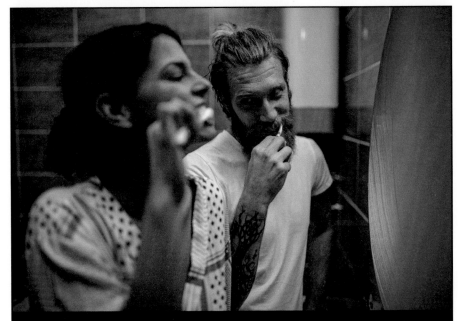

People living with someone with chronic hepatitis B should be careful not to share personal items that may have blood on them. Toothbrushes, for example, may have trace amounts of blood from breaks in the gums.

## Transmission

Hepatitis B is highly transmissible. It can survive outside of the body for at least seven days on a dry surface. Hepatitis B is passed from person to person through blood, semen, and vaginal secretions. It is usually passed through unprotected sexual contact including vaginal, anal, and oral sex. But people can contract hepatitis B through other nonsexual means. Any activity that transfers infected body fluids through the skin can transmit the virus.

A person with chronic hepatitis B may pass the disease to other people in their household through sharing toothbrushes, nail clippers, razors, or other objects that can have blood on them. As with other STIs, parents can pass the virus to their unborn children during pregnancy and delivery.

People getting tattooed, undergoing acupuncture treatment, or getting body parts pierced can contract hepatitis B if the same needle was previously used on an infected person. These activities generally occur in sterile environments, but clients should ensure their provider follows proper safety guidelines. Individuals who share hypodermic needles could also be exposed to hepatitis B.

People in health-care settings also have a higher risk of contracting hepatitis B due to regular exposure to body fluids. Health-care providers follow strict safety guidelines to prevent exposure, both to themselves and to their patients. US blood supplies are routinely screened for hepatitis B and C, and so transmission through blood transfusion is unlikely. Needles and syringes are stored in secure containers and sent to a medical waste management center for sterilization and disposal.

Hepatitis B cannot be transmitted through saliva, so it is not passed through coughing, sneezing, or kissing. It also cannot be spread by inanimate objects if those objects haven't touched blood.

## Symptoms

People infected with hepatitis B may be asymptomatic, or have no symptoms, but are still infectious. About two-thirds of those with hepatitis B antibodies in their blood never recall having the disease. For those who do show symptoms, these generally appear between one and four months after infection. Symptoms can include achy joints, extreme fatigue, loss of appetite, mild fever, abdominal pain, diarrhea and light-colored bowel movements, nausea and vomiting, jaundice, and dark urine.

Symptoms range from mild to severe and usually last about one to two months. The current treatment for people experiencing hepatitis B symptoms is supportive care, as most people return to full health on their own. About 90 to 95 percent of people who are infected recover completely and then have lifelong immunity from that strain of hepatitis. In rare cases, patients can experience liver failure and death shortly after infection.

Infected individuals who do not recover within six months are considered chronically infected. An estimated 880,000 to 1.89 million people in the United States have chronic hepatitis B, and up to two-thirds of them may not realize they have hepatitis B because they do not have any symptoms. If left untreated at birth, 90 percent of babies born with a hepatitis B infection will develop chronic hepatitis B.

One-third of people who are chronically infected develop chronic active hepatitis. It can lead to cirrhosis, or serious liver damage; liver cancer; and death. Two-thirds of those who are chronically infected have chronic persistent hepatitis and suffer mild inflammation of the liver. They are at some risk of developing cirrhosis and liver cancer, but their risk is not as great.

Chronically infected individuals are also carriers of the disease. This means they are contagious even though they show no outward symptoms of the virus. Although chronically infected individuals typically are infected for the rest of their lives, they sometimes recover.

## Diagnosis

A doctor may order blood work for a patient displaying physical symptoms. If tests show abnormal liver function, they may then order blood tests that specifically look for antibodies or antigens to confirm a hepatitis diagnosis. In rare cases of chronic hepatitis, a liver biopsy may be necessary. This procedure involves examining a small sample of liver tissue under a microscope. A biopsy can determine the stage of infection and the extent of damage.

Anyone who acquires hepatitis B should also be tested for hepatitis D, a blood-borne strain transmitted through needles and sexual contact. Hepatitis D uses hepatitis B to reproduce and survive and thus only infects people who have hepatitis B.

## Treatment

Hepatitis B is incurable, but it is also preventable. A safe and effective vaccine—three shots over the course of six months—has been available since 1982. The vaccine effectively eliminates the

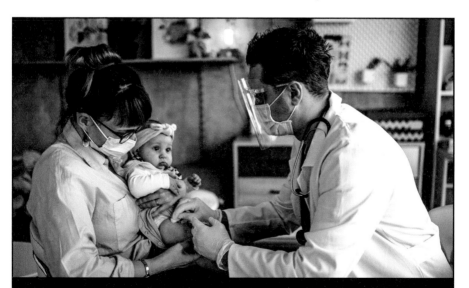

Health-care experts recommend that all infants receive their first dose of the hepatitis B vaccine at birth. A second dose is recommended at one to two months; the third dose can be scheduled after six months.

possibility of contracting the virus. Immunization against hepatitis B also protects against hepatitis D.

The CDC recommends that all babies be vaccinated against hepatitis B. Others who should be vaccinated include

- unvaccinated teens, particularly teens who are sexually active or who practice tattooing or body piercing
- children whose parents come from regions where chronic hepatitis B infection is common, such as Southeast Asia, Africa, the Amazon basin in South America, the Pacific Islands, and the Middle East
- people who use intravenous drugs
- nurses, doctors, dentists, laboratory workers, paramedics, and anyone else whose job exposes them to human blood
- partners of or anyone else who lives with someone with hepatitis B
- people who have multiple sexual partners
- prison inmates
- people receiving dialysis, a treatment that cleanses the patient's blood after the kidneys have failed

An unvaccinated person exposed to hepatitis B can get the vaccination series and a dose of hepatitis B antibodies that boosts the immune system for a short time. The two together offer some protection against infection. This method greatly reduces the likelihood of a pregnant person passing the virus onto their child. Infants are unlikely to acquire hepatitis B if they receive vaccinations and antibodies within twelve hours after birth.

If someone does contract hepatitis B, the infection usually goes away on its own. Doctors usually prescribe bed rest and plenty of fluids if symptoms appear. Hospitalization is unnecessary unless a person has other medical problems or is extremely ill.

People with chronic hepatitis infections sometimes benefit from treatment with injections of synthetic interferons, antiviral proteins that protect cells from infection by interfering with viral replication. Patients may be prescribed antiviral drugs to reduce or eliminate symptoms. However, the virus may develop a resistance to these medications.

People with chronic hepatitis B infection should be monitored for liver cancer. This monitoring involves regular ultrasounds and blood tests to check for liver damage.

People with liver failure from hepatitis B can extend their lives by receiving a liver transplant. Because of the scarcity of available livers, only a small number of hepatitis B patients receive liver transplants each year. Approximately eighteen hundred Americans die each year from a chronic hepatitis B infection. Those who receive a transplant must be careful to avoid reinfection.

There is a current push in medical research to find a cure for hepatitis B. The US National Institutes of Health (NIH) recently announced new funds for hepatitis research. But with hepatitis B affecting about 296 million people around the world, much more funding is needed. Timothy Block, a microbiologist from Pennsylvania who cofounded the Hepatitis B Foundation, says "Hepatitis B is completely overlooked and the funding is totally out of proportion to the problem and the need."

# CHAPTER 9

# WHY HAVEN'T STIs DISAPPEARED?

STIs continue to pose a threat to human health, even in the age of antibiotics and modern medicine. There are a variety of reasons including these:

## Lack of Information

Educating people about STIs has always been difficult. Many Americans believe that anything relating to sex is a private topic. Some have never been taught about sex and sexual health and don't want to reveal their ignorance. Some adults don't talk to their children about sexual matters because they believe that young people who are informed are more likely to be sexually active. This is false. Young people are equally as likely to be sexually active whether they have comprehensive sex education or not, so it is a better strategy to provide them with the information they need to be safe.

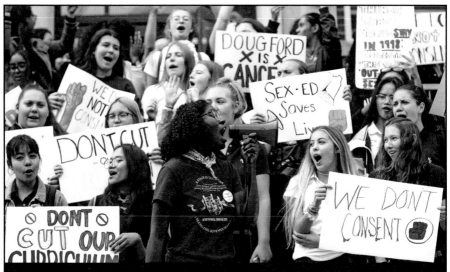

High school students throughout the province of Ontario, Canada, participated in a series of walkouts in September 2018. The students were protesting changes to the provincial health curriculum, which excluded mention of sexual orientation, consent, sexting, and other elements of comprehensive and inclusive sex education.

Sex education classes in schools sometimes offer comprehensive information about STIs, but these classes can be boring or preachy. Students may be turned off by how material is presented and tune it out. Some teens do not attend class regularly or drop out of school and miss the message altogether. Media messages about STIs are more attention-getting. But these can only give general advice rather than detailed, accurate information about preventing STIs or getting treatment for them.

## Embarrassment

Many people don't talk about STIs with their sexual partners because they are embarrassed. It is hard to discuss sex with someone you're trying to impress, someone you're not sure likes you, or someone you're afraid you might offend. STIs, which some people associate with promiscuity, are even more difficult to talk about. It's important to battle this stereotype—people can contract an STI from a single sexual partner or in some cases from nonsexual contact, and many people can have an STI without knowing it. If teens are sexually intimate with their partners before discussing one another's sexual history, it might be too late to protect their sexual health.

## Lack of Access to Health Care

People who live in poverty may not be able to afford visits to the doctor, or they may not have an easily accessible clinic when they need treatment. For this reason, they may not seek treatment even if they suspect they have an infection. Some marginalized groups that have experienced poor treatment from the medical system are suspicious of these institutions, and so they may stay away from health clinics that can provide information and treatment, even those that provide free services.

## Religious and Cultural Taboos

Religious beliefs and traditions that discourage or condemn premarital sex, promiscuity, and adultery sometimes also discourage discussions of STIs. Many religions preach that because teens should avoid sexual behavior altogether, they do not need to know about STIs and safer sex.

Some religious groups discourage the use of condoms because they believe that birth control is wrong. They feel that humans do not have the right to prevent conception and pregnancy.

In some cultural groups, women do not have the right to question their partner's sexual activities. They may not have the right to demand safer sex. These religious and cultural customs make controlling the spread of STIs more difficult.

While cultural and religious beliefs are personal, people from every cultural and religious background can be affected by STIs, so it is important to have the information to make health decisions that are right for you, whatever your sexual choices and beliefs may be.

## Media Messages

Many people hesitate to talk about sex. Yet music, movies, television, and the internet are filled with messages that sex is irresistible, trouble-free, and fun. Characters in many TV shows think about sex, joke about sex, and have casual sexual encounters. They don't much worry about the potential physical outcomes of their actions. In their storybook lives, they deal with romantic love and broken hearts. Yet they seldom, if ever, cope with the complications of an STI such as herpes or genital warts. The main message that comes across is that everyone is having sexual encounters, but nobody is worrying about the complications and responsibilities that go along with such encounters. Little to no communication is about the longer-term outcomes from sex, unless to lend drama or comedy to the story line, such as a character contracting an STI from an old partner, experiencing injuries from rough sex, or becoming pregnant after a single sexual encounter. This evasion does not present a complete picture of sexual health. In an era where many teens look to media for inspiration on how to live their lives, the omission of accurate information about or representations of sexual health risks can lead teens to mistakenly believe that there are no such risks.

# More Numerous Sexual Contacts

Americans tend to have multiple sexual contacts over the course of their lives. Most sexually active teens describe themselves as monogamous—they are having sex with only one person. But feelings and relationships can change rapidly. Someone who is monogamous can still have several partners in a relatively short period of time.

More sexual contact means there are more opportunities to transfer disease from one person to another. This is especially true when people do not take precautions to minimize the spread of STIs during sex. A common conception about sex is that it should be spontaneous, romantic, and passionate. Some people may feel guilty if they deliberately plan for it, or they may consider it promiscuous to prepare for sex by carrying around a condom. Neither of these is true. It is not promiscuous, nor is it unromantic, to protect yourself and your partner. Rather than turn your partner off, planning a sexual encounter with your partner can build anticipation and get you both in the mood. Your partner might find it sexy that you carry a condom with you. Reframing these activities as sexy for yourself and your partners helps reduce the stigma of talking about sex.

## Misplaced Trust

Teens might believe that trusting a partner is more important than asking questions and being careful about sex. But trust can be misplaced. Some people may lie about their sexual past to convince their partner to be intimate with them or because they are embarrassed about it. Someone might not know that they were

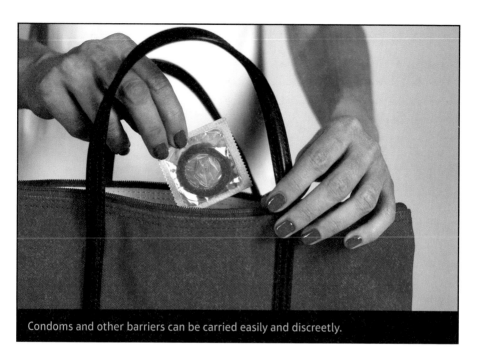

Condoms and other barriers can be carried easily and discreetly.

previously exposed to an STI and only learn after transmitting it to their current partner. Such situations can be harmful to or even end a relationship. A good idea before becoming sexually intimate with a partner is to get tested for STIs together. This can make sure that both partners are fully aware of the other's status before engaging in a sexual relationship.

## Alcohol and Drugs

Alcohol and drug use may lead someone to engage in sexual behavior that can increase the likelihood of transmitting or acquiring STIs. Substance use can impair judgment, which means that people might have unprotected sex and be less likely to consider the long-term complications of STIs. Individuals who choose to consume substances should keep this in mind. Keeping substance use low enough to avoid significant judgment impairment or ensuring that a friend is watching out for you are two ways to decrease risk when using substances.

## Denial

Despite the rising numbers of young people contracting STIs in the United States, many do not believe that they will acquire an STI. Some people might think they are not old enough or sexually active enough to contract an STI. Or they might mistakenly think that STIs affect only certain groups of people, such as LGBTQIA+ people, sex workers, people of low socioeconomic status, or people from different countries. But STIs can affect anyone.

# CHAPTER 10

# STI RISK REDUCTION

By doing research and taking proper precautions, anyone can lower, if not eliminate, the likelihood of either passing on or acquiring an STI.

## Abstinence

There is only one sure way to prevent transmitting or contracting an STI: total sexual abstinence. That means not engaging in sexual activity that involves genital contact with another person. Abstinence is a very personal decision, and everyone must decide on their own whether it is right for them. Many people choose abstinence for a variety of spiritual, emotional, and physical reasons. Some may choose to be abstinent on and off throughout their life. Anybody can be abstinent at any time, even if they have engaged in sexual activity before.

## SEXUAL PRESSURE

Setting boundaries can be hard, and a sexual partner may try to overstep the boundaries you set. Rape is the most obvious example of violently forcing someone beyond their sexual boundaries. But there are also subtle ways to take advantage of someone sexually. Verbal pressure is the most common and can be extremely compelling. Someone who is pressuring you might try put-downs: "You're weird. Nobody waits anymore." Or reassurances: "Don't worry, I'm clean." Or casting doubt on your relationship: "Don't you love me?"

Verbal coercion, just like physical coercion, meets the legal definition of rape. Nobody should ever be verbally pressuring you to engage in a sexual activity that you are not comfortable with.

If you are being verbally pressured, you can prepare yourself with good responses. For example, if someone is trying to reassure you that they don't have an STI, you can say, "For all you know, I may have an STI. Let's both be safe rather than sorry."

Some people object to using condoms or other barriers, claiming that they are too much trouble, are too embarrassing to buy, or are not perfectly reliable. But for

## Safer Sex

For those who do not choose abstinence, they can reduce the likelihood of contracting an STI. It's smart to have a conversation about your sexual boundaries and expectations with your partner most, the effort is worth it to protect oneself and their partner against the potential transmission of STIs. And sex may be more enjoyable when partners are not fearful of becoming pregnant or acquiring an STI. A person should always have a condom or another barrier if there is any chance of having sex, and they should be prepared to refuse to have sex if a partner refuses to use a barrier.

If you are ever in a sexual situation where you feel unsafe, remove yourself from the situation as quickly as possible. Excuse yourself to the bathroom and call a friend, a parent, or 911.

If you experience sexual assault, sexual harassment, domestic violence, or any sexual experience in which you felt unsafe or your boundaries weren't respected, you can call the National Sexual Assault Hotline at (800) 656-4673. The National Sexual Violence Resource Center also offers online resources about sexual violence. If you suspect you may be in an abusive relationship, the love is respect helpline at (866) 331-9474 is a good resource.

If you experience sexual violence, it is always a good idea to seek mental health services. Some people think they are unaffected by the experience, but many find it helps to talk with a mental health professional.

before getting physical. That way, you can minimize pressure or confusion that may arise in the moment. This conversation may involve planning ahead for certain situations, such as if a partner starts showing symptoms of an STI. Discussing your sexual history at this point can also help you understand and reduce the likelihood of transmission during sex. Many people get tested for STIs regularly and communicate their results with their partners.

Talking about sex can feel awkward or embarrassing. Here are some guidelines that can make discussing sex more comfortable:

- Pick a public place to talk where you will not be disturbed or overheard.
- Don't have discussions while under the influence of alcohol or drugs.
- Have an opening line that will ease into the discussion. For instance, begin with "This is a little embarrassing to talk about" or "This is hard to bring up." That gets the awkwardness out in the open and prepares your partner. Then say something like this: "We really seem to like each other, and I think we should talk about how far we're willing to go physically." If you're not sure that the time is right, you can start with, "I have something a little embarrassing to talk about. Is it okay if I bring it up now?" If your partner refuses to discuss the topic, then you should make it clear that you are not ready to become physically intimate.
- Talk about your own attitudes and feelings. Begin your sentences with "I think . . ." or "I feel . . ." Encourage your partner to express their feelings too. Recognize and respect that they may want different things from a sexually intimate relationship than you do. Try to listen without being judgmental and communicate your beliefs without preaching—and expect the same in return.

- Be specific. Simply saying that you don't want to go "too far" can lead to misunderstandings. Try to explain in more detail how intimate you are willing to be.
- You don't have to make an immediate decision. You or your partner might need a few days to sort out your feelings. Keep lines of communication open, and try to be available when your partner is ready to revisit your discussion.

If you have established boundaries, discussed your sexual history, and decided to be sexually intimate, you will want to talk about birth control options as well as ways to minimize the transmission of STIs. Although condoms do not offer protection from all sores and

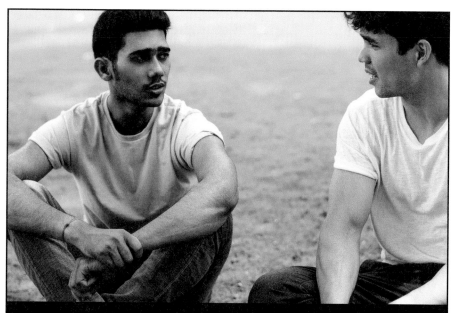

Good communication is an important part of any healthy relationship. Being open and honest can make it easier to deal with conflict and build stronger partnerships.

lesions or from viral shedding, using a new condom for every sexual encounter significantly lowers the rate of STI transmission between partners. Condoms are what's known as a barrier and can significantly reduce the likelihood of acquiring an STI during sex. They are also 95 percent effective in preventing pregnancy.

Condoms can be purchased in a grocery, drug, or discount store, and no prescription is necessary. Condoms are also sometimes available for purchase in public restrooms. People can use external condoms, which go over the penis, or internal condoms, which are inserted into the vagina. To be effective in preventing STI infection and pregnancy, store and use condoms according to their directions. Most condom failures are a result of not storing them or putting them on properly. Additionally, using oil-based lubricants can damage latex condoms. Natural condoms, known as skins or lambskins, are more porous than latex condoms and do not provide adequate protection against STIs.

Another barrier option is the dental dam, a thin sheet of latex or polyurethane. Dental dams provide protection from STIs when sexual contact is occurring between one person's mouth and another person's vagina or anus. As with condoms, using dental dams according to their instructions and using a new one for each sexual encounter can reduce the likelihood of STI transmission. Dental dams are not as easy to find as condoms. While they may be available at some drugstores, the easiest option for many people is to order them online.

## Getting Tested for STIs

Usually, people with STIs do not experience any symptoms. Testing is one way to make sure of your status. Knowing the results can also offer peace of mind for sexual partners. People who are sexually active and meet any of the following criteria should talk to a health-care provider about being tested for STIs:

- had sex without barriers with a partner and don't know if that person has an STI
- had a new sexual partner within the past sixty days
- had more than two sexual partners in the past six months
- had sexual contact with someone with an STI or have contracted an STI in the past twelve months
- are pregnant or planning to become pregnant
- are not consistently using barriers with new partners
- have been diagnosed with PID or infections of the urethra, epididymis, or prostate

# Guidelines to Lower Your Risk

People can take additional steps to reduce the likelihood of acquiring or transmitting an STI. These include

- getting vaccinated for hepatitis B and HPV
- avoiding contact with the body fluids of someone whose health and sexual history are unknown to you
- ensuring you and your partners are tested regularly
- never having sex while under the influence of drugs or alcohol
- never sharing needles or having sex with someone who shares needles of any kind

# CHAPTER 11

# LIVING WITH A CHRONIC STI

Individuals can do several things if they discover they have a chronic STI such as herpes, hepatitis B, or HIV. These include being as knowledgeable as possible about STIs, getting necessary treatments, maintaining a healthy lifestyle, and connecting with supportive friends and family for emotional and practical help.

## Be Informed

People living with a chronic STI can take control of their health by finding out everything they can about their disease. For instance, if they have genital herpes, they can learn to recognize the prodromal symptoms that may signal an upcoming outbreak. Pinpointing and avoiding foods or situations that trigger outbreaks are also key coping skills. Individuals with HIV can learn about ways to build up their immune system. They can ask their doctor about new types of treatments and new medications.

Someone who has an STI that causes blisters or sores is more likely to contract other STIs. For instance, during a herpes outbreak, a person can more easily contract HIV if exposed. Informing sexual partners of any health considerations and practicing safer sex are vital to ensuring positive and healthy sexual encounters.

# Get Regular Medical Checkups

Regular medical checkups are important for people with chronic STIs. Early detection and diagnosis can lessen the odds of future complications. For instance, current recommendations by the US Preventive Services Task Force recommend that all young people with a cervix, beginning at the age of twenty-one, receive screening Pap tests every three years. If a person has an abnormal Pap test, they should get Pap tests yearly until either their Pap tests return to normal or the cervical abnormalities require further intervention.

A physician can be an excellent source of information about ways to cope with a chronic STI. When meeting with a doctor, bring a list of your concerns and questions to avoid forgetting or overlooking something while you are in the doctor's office.

For those who cannot afford to go to a doctor, many communities have health departments, infectious disease clinics, STI clinics, women's health clinics, or family-planning clinics where testing and treatment are free or low cost and where your personal information is confidential. The national STI hotline of the CDC at (800) 232-4636 can help you access these types of treatment centers in your area.

Drugs that are prescribed to treat an STI should be taken as directed. This may mean taking a pill at a certain time of day or avoiding certain foods while taking certain medications. It is

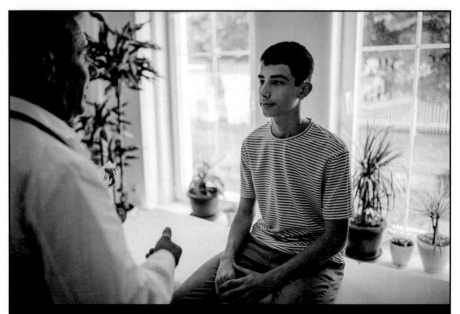

Patients can work with a doctor to come up with a plan to manage a chronic STI through drug therapy, counseling, and alternative treatment options.

important not to skip doses, combine doses, or stop taking medicine too soon. Doctors, pharmacists, and other health-care providers can answer patients' questions. Follow-up appointments can ensure that drug side effects are not serious and that prescribed drugs are working as they should.

## Adopt a Healthy Lifestyle

A strong immune system is a person's best defense against outbreaks of herpes or the progression of HIV or AIDS. Maintaining a healthy lifestyle will help keep the immune system strong. A healthy lifestyle includes eating a balanced diet, getting enough sleep, exercising regularly, avoiding smoking and vaping, avoiding

# WHAT IF I WANT TO HAVE CHILDREN?

People who have chronic STIs can still have children, but they must ensure that they do not transmit an STI to their children. Before becoming pregnant, check with a doctor. Certain medications that are used to control symptoms of STIs can be dangerous for a developing fetus. A doctor may suggest changes in treatment if a person with an STI is pregnant or nursing a baby.

Health-care providers follow guidelines to reduce the possibility of prenatal transmission. Proper treatment can dramatically reduce the likelihood of passing HIV to a fetus during pregnancy. Antiviral medication can prevent an outbreak of herpes that may be transmitted to a baby at birth. If a patient is having a herpes outbreak when they are ready to give birth, their doctor may opt to perform a cesarean section to prevent the baby from acquiring an infection during a vaginal delivery. In this operation, the doctor delivers the baby through an incision in the abdomen and uterus.

the misuse of alcohol and drugs, and pursuing stress-reducing activities.

## Find Someone to Talk To

People who learn that they have an STI may feel a range of emotions, including fear, depression, and shame. The feelings can be even more complex if they contracted the STI from someone they were

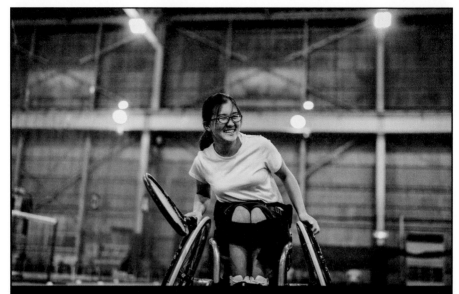

A 2017 study found that moderate exercise improved the quality of life of females with HIV. Results showed improvement in all measured parameters, including physical, psychological, and social well-being.

emotionally intimate with and trusted. Feelings of betrayal, anger, sadness, and frustration are normal reactions. They might feel anxious and guilty knowing that they could transmit an STI to their sexual partners, or that they may have transmitted it to their previous sexual partners. They may be afraid they will be rejected when they tell a new partner about their infection. Some people may decide to keep the news a secret, including from their parents, closest friends, or even sexual partners. But being open about your health and getting help are key to managing STIs.

Family and friends are often the strongest source of support. They can provide valuable guidance and encouragement. Many teens fear and put off telling parents or guardians, convinced that they will be judgmental, harsh, and unreasonable. Usually, caretakers want to help. Most will be understanding and willing to do what they can.

But some parents and other family members may not be available or supportive. Or they might need additional assistance. Health-care workers, counselors, trusted adults at school or in some places of worship, hotlines, and online resources can provide comfort, insights, and encouragement. Young volunteers who staff hotlines and community health clinics can be particularly helpful to teens with STIs. A variety of national and local support groups can also help teens.

## To Tell or Not to Tell?

There can be a lot of fear around disclosing an STI to a current or potential partner. It may feel awkward or uncomfortable, especially if sexual health is not something that has been a part of your discussions before. You may be worried about how your partner will react. Maybe that they will end the relationship or tell others about your diagnosis or try to make you feel guilty for having contracted an STI.

Contracting an STI can happen to anybody, and for many people it is a normal part of the human experience, like getting food poisoning or breaking a bone. While it can be tempting to avoid telling your partner, it is always better to tell them about your diagnosis and any treatments you are taking. Sexual consent should be clearly and freely communicated. By not giving them all the information, you are depriving your partner of the ability to make an informed decision about their own sexual health and violating their consent. Many relationships are based on trust, and by electing not to disclose an STI, you take away some of that trust that is very difficult to rebuild.

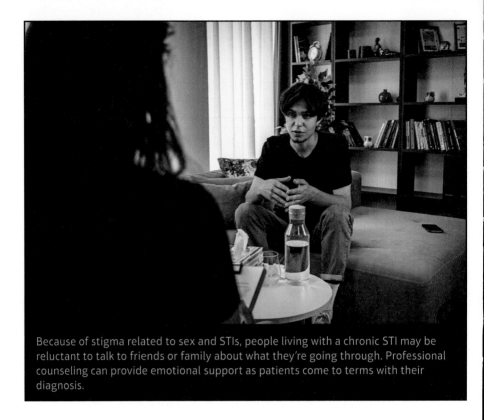

Because of stigma related to sex and STIs, people living with a chronic STI may be reluctant to talk to friends or family about what they're going through. Professional counseling can provide emotional support as patients come to terms with their diagnosis.

Most STIs can be cured with current medical treatment, and all can be managed. You and your partner have a lot of options in sexual intimacy and transmission prevention.

If you are nervous about speaking with your partner, many physicians or other medical professionals will allow you to bring your partner or partners into their office so that all of you can speak together about your diagnosis and what it means for the future of the relationship and your sexual health. This can make the conversation easier while ensuring that a health-care professional is present to dispel any myths or prejudices about STIs and present up-to-date information about how to best manage and treat STIs.

# How Do I Tell My Partner?

Telling a sexual partner—especially a new partner—about a chronic STI can be very difficult. Someone with an STI can minimize discomfort and embarrassment when breaking the news by preparing what they will say in advance.

These guidelines, like those for talking about sex in general, can help make the discussion a little easier:

- If this is the beginning of a relationship, get to know your partner first. It is not necessary to reveal that you have an STI on the first date, although you should tell your partner before becoming sexually intimate. If you are already in a sexual relationship, you should tell your partner as soon as possible.
- Pick a public place to talk where you will not be disturbed or overheard. Talk face-to-face if possible. It's sometimes hard, if not impossible, to gauge a person's emotions through a DM or even a phone call. Some good opening lines could be "I think I can trust you, so I'd like to tell you something very personal," or "I need to let you know something about me. It may or may not be a big deal to you."
- Have your discussion free of the influence of alcohol or drugs.
- Start your discussion in a nonsexual atmosphere. Don't have your conversation just as you are beginning to have sex or immediately afterward. Instead, choose a time when your thinking is clear and focused.

- Take a calm, matter-of-fact approach. The more positive you are, the more likely your partner will be calm and positive too. Be open and honest, and answer all questions. Convey to your partner that you know a lot about your STI and how to deal with it to keep you both healthy.
- Give your partner time to adjust. Remember how you felt when you found out you had an infection. Don't force a reaction or decision immediately. Avoid becoming angry or judgmental. Treat your partner the way you would like to be treated in the same situation.
- If your partner is accepting of your news, talk about the options—abstinence, using barriers during sex, having forms of sex that are less likely to cause transmission, or treatment plans that mitigate or eliminate any possibility of transmission. Explain how your STI can be spread so your partner can take necessary precautions. Encourage your partner to visit a doctor for any necessary testing.

Sometimes, news of your STI may be something that your sexual partner can't deal with. That person may choose to walk away from the relationship. If that happens, support from your family and friends or from a therapist can help you process your feelings. Remember that you did the right thing by sharing your news and that you are in charge of your sexual health. Many partners will be very understanding and accepting. If the two of you navigate sexual health together, you may find that the relationship has grown stronger.

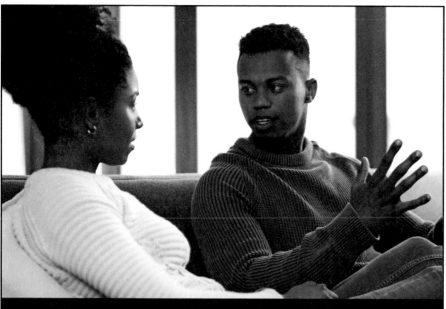
Having a calm, straightforward, and honest discussion about STIs can help both partners navigate how best to manage their sexual and emotional health.

## Reach Out to Others

Teens who are living with a chronic STI may want to help others learn about prevention and control. Teens can become involved, both at school and in the community.

- In health classes, help ensure that the most up-to-date information on STIs is presented. Do some research and give a report on the subject, get permission to create a bulletin board, or line up a special guest speaker.
- Work with school administrators and parent groups to ensure that students are aware of available

information about STI prevention. Help counselors research and order pamphlets and brochures to give to interested students. Help schedule a speaker who will come to the school and give a presentation at an assembly. School administrators must work within state and local sex education guidelines when presenting information on STIs. Some teens may attend an abstinence-only school district, for example. There, education about STI prevention—through any means other than abstinence—is not permitted.

- Write an editorial or an article for a local newspaper or an online support group about STIs.
- Work with health-care groups in the community. A teen clinic or a teen hotline may need volunteers and can offer training.

## Understanding Transmission and Treatment

Researchers, doctors, and public health officials are working to find health solutions for people with STIs. New therapies and drugs to better treat STIs are being tested and approved, and the research to find cures is ongoing. While this is encouraging, prevention continues to be the best way to stem the spread of STIs. As people continually become better educated about STIs, they also become better able to protect themselves and those they care about.

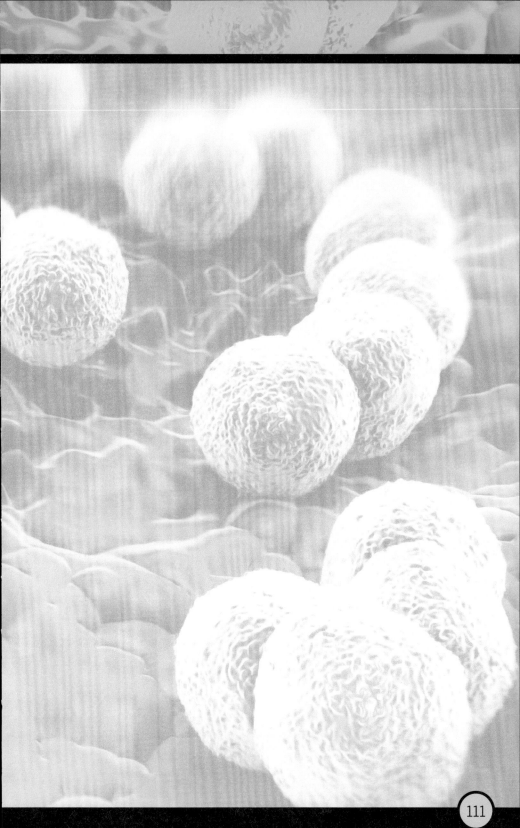

# GLOSSARY

**abstinence:** not doing or having something, such as sexual relations

**acquired immunodeficiency syndrome (AIDS):** a disease caused by HIV in which the immune system is severely compromised and makes a person vulnerable to infection and illness

**antibody:** a protein produced by the immune system to fight off infection

**antigen:** a protein, chemical, or bacteria on the surface of an organism that stimulates the production of antibodies

**antiretroviral (ARV):** a drug to treat infections caused by retroviruses, such as HIV

**anus:** the opening at the lower end of the large intestine through which waste is released

**asymptomatic:** a person who does not show symptoms of an infection or disease

**autoinoculation:** an infection caused by a disease that has spread from another part of the body

**carrier:** an infected person who may be asymptomatic but who can pass infection to others

**cervix:** the part of the uterus that opens to the vagina

**chancre (SHAN-ker):** a painless, highly infectious ulcer that is the first symptom of primary syphilis

**chlamydia (kluh-MID-ee-ah):** an STI caused by the bacterium *Chlamydia trachomatis* (*C. trachomatis*) that can infect the urinary-genital area, the anal area, and sometimes the eyes, throat, and lungs

**clitoris:** the female organ of sexual arousal

**colposcopy:** a procedure where the vagina is examined using a colposcope, a magnifying and photographic instrument

**condom:** a latex sheath worn over the penis or in the vagina during sex to prevent pregnancy and STIs

**deoxyribonucleic acid (DNA):** a nucleic acid or group of nucleic acids that makes up the genes of all living organisms

**dissemination:** spreading over or through a large area

**ectopic pregnancy:** the implantation and development of a fertilized egg outside of the uterus

**enzyme-linked immunosorbent assay (ELISA):** a diagnostic test in which antigens or antibodies are detected by an enzyme that converts a colorless substance into a colored product

**epidemic:** an outbreak of disease that spreads more widely or more quickly among a group of people than would normally be expected

**epididymis:** a duct through which sperm pass from the testicle to the vas deferens

**fallopian tube:** one of two narrow tubes through which eggs pass from the ovary to the uterus

**fetus:** an unborn human offspring after eight weeks of development

**genitals:** exterior reproductive organs

**genital wart:** an irregular skin growth caused by the human papillomavirus (HPV)

**gonorrhea:** an STI caused by the bacterium *Neisseria gonorrhoeae* (*N. gonorrhoeae*), which produces genital infections and can also infect the mouth, the throat, and the anal area

**hepatitis B:** a virus commonly passed through an exchange of infected body fluids including blood, semen, and vaginal secretions

**herpes:** an STI that is part of a viral family that can cause cold sores, chicken pox, shingles, and mononucleosis

**highly active antiretroviral therapy (HAART):** a powerful combination of ARVs prescribed to treat HIV and AIDS

**human immunodeficiency virus (HIV):** a retrovirus that attacks the immune system

**human papillomavirus (HPV):** viruses that cause warts on hands, feet, and genitals as well as cervical cancer

**immune system:** a complex body system that aids the body in fighting off disease

**immunity:** being able to resist a particular disease

**infertility:** unable to reproduce

**intravenous:** administered into a vein, usually with a needle

**labia:** fleshy folds that surround the opening of the vagina

**lesion:** any kind of abnormality of a tissue or organ due to a disease or injury

**monogamous:** having a sexual relationship with only one partner at a time

**neurosyphilis:** an infection of the nervous system by *T. pallidum*, the bacterium that causes syphilis

**opportunistic infection:** a condition caused by a microorganism that may not normally cause disease but that becomes life-threatening when a host's immunity is impaired

**ovary:** one of two reproductive organs that produces eggs and hormones

**Pap test:** a test to detect a precancerous or cancerous condition of the cervix

**pathogen:** an agent such as a bacterium or virus that causes disease

**pelvic inflammatory disease (PID):** an infection of the ovaries, fallopian tubes, and uterus that can lead to infertility

**penis:** the reproductive organ that discharges urine and semen

**polymerase chain reaction (PCR):** the technique by which a small fragment of genetic material can be rapidly duplicated to produce multiple copies

**prodrome:** a period during which symptoms appear that can indicate an upcoming outbreak of herpes

**prostate:** a reproductive gland lying below the bladder that produces part of the fluid in semen

**retrovirus:** a family of viruses with a unique mode of replication

**ribonucleic acid (RNA):** a nucleic acid or group of nucleic acids associated with the control of cellular chemical activity

**safer sex:** taking precautions to reduce the likelihood of STI transmission or pregnancy during sexual activity

**scrotum:** the loose sac of skin and muscles that holds the testicles

**semen:** a fluid containing sperm

**seminal vesicle:** the reproductive gland that produces semen

**sexually transmitted infection (STI):** also known as a sexually transmitted disease (STD) or venereal disease (VD); a bacterial or viral infection that can be passed from person to person during sexual contact

**shedding:** when the herpes virus is present on the skin and can be easily passed to others

**sperm:** male reproductive cells

**syndrome:** the symptomatic phase of a herpes outbreak

**syphilis:** an STI caused by the bacterium *Treponema pallidum* (*T. pallidum*) that can affect virtually every part of the body

**testicle:** the reproductive organ that produces sperm and the hormone testosterone

**ulcer:** a slow-healing sore

**urethra:** the tube that transports urine out of the body

**uterus:** the reproductive organ in which a fetus develops

**vagina:** also known as the birth canal; the muscular tube connecting the uterus to the outside of the body

**vas deferens:** the duct through which sperm is carried from the epididymis to the urethra

**vulva:** external sex organs including the clitoris, the vaginal opening, and the labia

**Western blot test:** a diagnostic test that looks for antibodies to infectious agents such as herpes and HIV

**yeast infection:** a fungal infection in the vagina, the mouth, or other parts of the body that causes irritation or other symptoms

# SOURCE NOTES

30  "Since the discovery . . . of existing [ones].": Chris Furniss, quoted in Conrad Duncan, "Scientists Discover New Approach to Fighting Antibiotic Resistance," Imperial College London, February 24, 2022, https://www.imperial.ac.uk/news/234060/scientists -discover-approach-fighting-antibiotic-resistance/.

31  "It is possible . . . currently available antibiotics.": Furniss.

59  "So much has . . . restrictions and criminalization.": Lawrence Gostin, "How AIDS Brought Global Health to the World Political Stage," Conversation, February 18, 2016, https://theconversation .com/how-aids-brought-global-health-to-the-world-political -stage-54415.

75–76  "Several countries which . . . of cervical cancer.": Douglas R. Lowy, quoted in Alana Hippensteele, "NCI Acting Director: Equitable Precision Medicine Requires Concerted Implementation Efforts," *Pharmacy Times*, September 29, 2022, https://www .pharmacytimes.com/view/nci-acting-director-equitable -precision-medicine-requires-concerted-implementation-efforts.

85  "Hepatitis B is . . . and the need.": Timothy Block, quoted in Jon Cohen, "The Push Is on to Cure Hepatitis B, a Long-Overlooked Scourge of Millions," *Science*, November 29, 2018, https:// www.science.org/content/article/push-cure-hepatitis-b-long -overlooked-scourge-millions.

# SELECTED BIBLIOGRAPHY

"Adolescents and Young Adults." Centers for Disease Control and Prevention. Accessed November 21, 2022. https://www.cdc.gov/std/life-stages -populations/adolescents-youngadults.htm.

"Basic Statistics." Centers for Disease Control and Prevention. Last updated June 21, 2022. https://www.cdc.gov/hiv/basics/statistics.html.

"Chlamydia—CDC Detailed Fact Sheet." Centers for Disease Control and Prevention. Last updated April 12, 2022. https://www.cdc.gov/std/chlamydia /stdfact-chlamydia-detailed.htm.

"11 Facts about Teens and STDs." DoSomething. Accessed June 15, 2022. https://www.dosomething.org/us/facts/11-facts-about-teens-and-std s#:~:text=1%20in%204%20teens%20contract,STD%20other%20than%20 HIV%2FAIDS.

"Genital Herpes—CDC Detailed Fact Sheet." Centers for Disease Control and Prevention. Last updated July 22, 2022. https://www.cdc.gov/std/herpes /stdfact-herpes-detailed.htm#ref2.

"Genital HPV Infection—Basic Fact Sheet." Centers for Disease Control and Prevention. Last updated April 12, 2022. https://www.cdc.gov/std/hpv /stdfact-hpv.htm.

"Gonorrhea—CDC Detailed Fact Sheet." Centers for Disease Control and Prevention. Last updated April 12, 2022. https://www.cdc.gov/std/gonorrhea /stdfact-gonorrhea-detailed.htm.

"Hepatitis B Questions and Answers for Health Professionals." Centers for Disease Control and Prevention. Last updated March 30, 2022. https://www .cdc.gov/hepatitis/hbv/hbvfaq.htm#b16.

"HIV Basics." Centers for Disease Control and Prevention. Last updated November 4, 2022. https://www.cdc.gov/hiv/basics/index.html.

"HIV Prevention." Centers for Disease Control and Prevention. Last updated June 1, 2021. https://www.cdc.gov/hiv/basics/prevention.html.

"HIV Testing." Centers for Disease Control and Prevention. Accessed November 21, 2022. https://www.cdc.gov/hiv/basics/testing.html.

"HIV Transmission." Centers for Disease Control and Prevention. Last updated October 28, 2020. https://www.cdc.gov/hiv/basics/transmission.html.

"Living with HIV." Centers for Disease Control and Prevention. Last updated May 20, 2021. https://www.cdc.gov/hiv/basics/livingwithhiv/index.html.

"Reported STDs Reach All-Time High for 6th Consecutive Year: More Than 2.5 Million Cases of Chlamydia, Gonorrhea, and Syphilis Reported in 2019." Centers for Disease Control and Prevention, April 13, 2021. https://www.cdc .gov/media/releases/2021/p0413-stds.html.

"Sexually Transmitted Infections (STIs)." World Health Organization, August 22, 2022. https://www.who.int/news-room/fact-sheets/detail/sexually -transmitted-infections-(stis).

"Syphilis—CDC Fact Sheet (Detailed)." Centers for Disease Control and Prevention. Last updated April 12, 2022. https://www.cdc.gov/std/syphilis /stdfact-syphilis-detailed.htm.

# RESOURCES

American Sexual Health Association (ASHA)
https://ashasexualhealth.org/
ASHA offers reliable, science-based, and stigma-free resources and information about STIs and sexual health.

Centers for Disease Control and Prevention (CDC) STI Hotline
https://www.cdc.gov/std/
(800) 232-4636
The CDC hotline and web page provide key resources about STI prevention and treatment.

HIV.gov
https://www.hiv.gov/
This website, managed by the US Department of Health & Human Services, outlines the federal response to the HIV epidemic and provides information on how to get tested, find services, and get a prescription for PrEP.

love is respect
https://www.loveisrespect.org/
(866) 331-9474
This national resource seeks to disrupt and prevent intimate partner violence. The site, in addition to offering a call, chat, and texting hotline, provides inclusive and equitable education for young people who have questions or concerns about their romantic and sexual relationships.

National Sexual Assault Hotline
https://www.rainn.org/get-help
(800) 656-4673
The Rape, Abuse & Incest National Network (RAINN) partners with more than one thousand local sexual assault service providers across the country to connect survivors with the help they need.

National Sexual Violence Resource Center
https://nsvrc.org/
The NSVRC offers research and tools for advocates working to end sexual harassment, assault, and abuse. The site provides a directory of organizations and local programs that can help and support survivors.

Planned Parenthood
https://plannedparenthood.org/
Planned Parenthood offers information and resources about STIs, safer sex, relationships, and more. The site includes a page dedicated to teen health and wellness.

# FURTHER READING

## Books for Young Adults

Honders, Christine. *The Dangers of Sexually Transmitted Diseases*. San Diego: Lucent Books, 2017.

Mirk, Sarah. *You Do You: Figuring Out Your Body, Dating, and Sexuality*. Minneapolis: Twenty-First Century Books, 2019.

Park, Ina. *Strange Bedfellows: Adventures in the Science, History, and Surprising Secrets of STDs*. New York: Flatiron Books, 2021.

Parrish, Jacqueline. *Coping with Sexually Transmitted Diseases*. New York: Rosen Young Adult, 2020.

Strehle Hartman, Ashley. *Teens and STDs*. San Diego: ReferencePoint, 2019.

Sycamore, Mattilda Bernstein, ed. *Between Certain Death and a Possible Future: Queer Writing on Growing Up with the AIDS Crisis*. Vancouver, BC: Arsenal Pulp, 2021.

## Books for Parents and Family Members

Quinn, Paul. *Sexually Transmitted Diseases: Your Questions Answered*. Santa Barbara, CA: Greenwood, 2018.

Rice, Daniel. *The Essential Sex Education Book for Parents: Guided Conversations to Have with Your Tweens and Teens*. Emeryville, CA: Rockridge, 2022.

## Websites

"Adolescent Sexual Health." National Coalition of STD Directors, August 28, 2017. https://www.ncsddc.org/project/ash/.
This site is a resource for teens to learn more about STIs and public health for adolescents.

Anzilotti, Amy. "How Do I Get Checked for STDs without My Parents Knowing?" Kidshealth.org, October 2018. https://kidshealth.org/en/teens/stds-check.html.
This information page includes tips on how to seek completely confidential STI services.

Bologna, Caroline. "How to Talk to Your Teen about STIs in a Helpful, Not Awkward Way." HuffPost, November 20, 2019. https://www.huffpost.com /entry/how-to-talk-to-teens-about--stis_l_5dd44d9be4b0e29d727af19f. Conversations about sex and STIs can be uncomfortable or awkward. Sex educators provide tips on how parents can have a supportive and stigma-free talk about STIs and safer sex with their teens.

"Chlamydia." Cleveland Clinic. Last reviewed November 1, 2021. https:// my.clevelandclinic.org/health/diseases/4023--chlamydia. Cleveland Clinic is a nonprofit academic medical center involved in health research and education. Their web page on chlamydia outlines prevention, symptoms, diagnosis, treatment options, and other common topics.

Gillespie, Susan. "Testing for Sexually Transmitted Infections (STIs)." American Academy of Pediatrics, January 2, 2022. https://www.healthychildren.org /English/health-issues/conditions/sexually-transmitted/Pages/Diagnostic -Testing-for-Sexually-Transmitted-Infections.aspx. Gillespie, a pediatrician specializing in HIV care for infants, children, and adolescents, provides parents with a thorough explanation of diagnostic testing for several STIs.

"HIV by Group." Centers for Disease Control and Prevention, April 14, 2022. https://www.cdc.gov/hiv/group/index.html. HIV can affect anyone, regardless of their age, gender, sexual orientation, or race. This information page highlights the challenges that different demographics face when preventing and treating HIV, as well as how the CDC is working to address those challenges.

Mandriota, Morgan. "9 Tips for Coping with a Positive STI Diagnosis." PsychCentral. Last reviewed March 7, 2022. https://psychcentral.com/health /tips-for-coping-with-positive-sti-diagnosis. Many people seek mental health resources after testing positive for an STI. PsychCentral offers a guide on different ways that people cope with an STI diagnosis.

Pierce, Jenelle Marie. "Living with an STI/STD—Reflecting on Stigma." STI Project. Last updated July 29, 2021. https://thestiproject.com/living-with -an-std-reflecting-on-the-week/. Jenelle Marie Pierce, executive director for the STI Project, writes about her past and present experiences with STI stigma in a blog post for the organization.

"Positively You!" Maricopa County Public Health. Accessed November 21, 2022. https://positivelyyouaz.com/.
Discover more about what it means to live with and manage STIs by watching videos from real people. This site, sponsored by the public health department in Maricopa County, Arizona, also provides information on local services and community partners.

Santhakumar, Sasha. "What to Know about HIV Risk among Transgender Women." Medical News Today, August 9, 2021. https://www .medicalnewstoday.com/articles/hiv-in-transgender-women.
Transgender women have an increased risk of contracting HIV. This article outlines some of the factors that contribute to this higher risk as well as prevention tips.

"Sexually Transmitted Diseases (STDs)." Centers for Disease Control and Prevention, January 13, 2022. https://www.cdc.gov/std/healthcomm/fact_ sheets.htm.
The CDC offers basic fact sheets to answer frequently asked questions about STIs in plain, accessible language. They also provide more detailed fact sheets for physicians and people who have more specific questions about infections and diseases.

Toronto Planned Parenthood. "Telling Your Partner You Have an STI." Teen Health Source. Last updated November 2022. https://teenhealthsource.com/stisetc /telling-partner-sti/.
Teen Health Source is a sexual health information resource created by Planned Parenthood in Toronto, Canada. This page addresses concerns about disclosing one's STI status to a sexual partner, ideas for breaking the ice around STIs, and recommendations for dealing with negative reactions to disclosure.

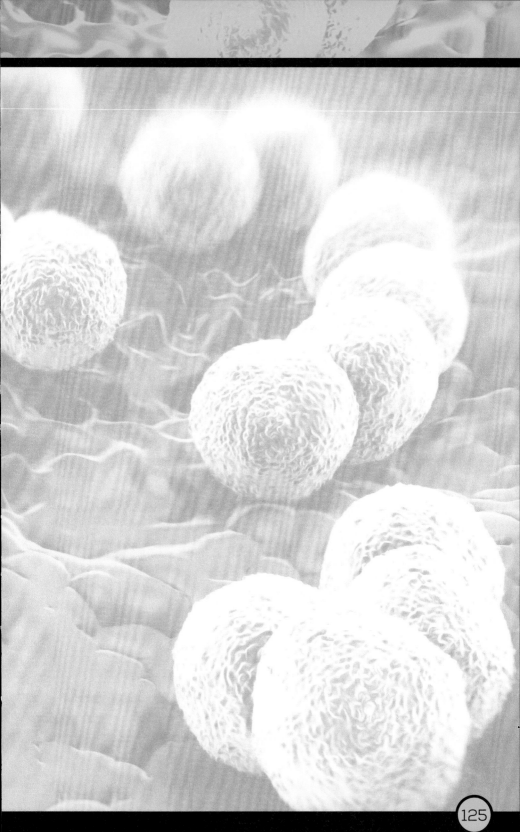

# INDEX

## ABOUT THE AUTHORS

Diane Yancey is the author of *Tuberculosis* and *Eating Disorders* as well as several other nonfiction titles for young people. She lives in western Washington.

Tabitha Moriarty is a medical student living in Atlanta, Georgia.

## PHOTO ACKNOWLEDGMENTS

Image credits: Prostock-studio/Shutterstock, p. 7; Maniki_rus/Shutterstock, p. 22; Laura Westlund/Independent Picture Service, pp. 11, 14; apichsn/iStockphoto/Getty Images/, p. 17; FatCamera/Getty Images, p. 19; SDI Productions/E+/Getty Images, p. 24; Teeramet Thanomkiat/EyeEm/Getty Images, p. 27; mikimad/E+/Getty Images, p. 32; CNRI/Science Source, p. 36; myibean/iStock/Getty Images, p. 43; Carol Yepes/Moment/Getty Images, p. 45; Peter Dressel/Tetra Images/Getty Images, p. 50; Science Source, p. 52; IM Vector Studio/Shutterstock, p. 53; nito/Alamy Stock Photo, p. 64; Catherine Falls Commercial/Getty Images, p. 67; VioletaStoimenova/Getty Images, p. 69; anastas/Getty Images, p. 75; Brian van der Brug/Los Angeles Times/Getty Images, p. 77; bernardbodo/Getty Images, p. 80; hobo_018/Getty Images, p. 83; Randy Risling/Toronto Star/Getty Images, p. 87; MangoStar_Studio/Getty Images, p. 97; South_agency/Getty Images, p. 102; ©2019 Kohei Hara/Getty Images, p. 104; Phynart Studio/Getty Images, p. 106; Dean Mitchell/Getty Images, p. 109. Backgrounds: MikeDotta/Shutterstock; Peddalanka Ramesh Babu/Shutterstock.

Cover: MikeDotta/Shutterstock; Peddalanka Ramesh Babu/Shutterstock.